AF376709

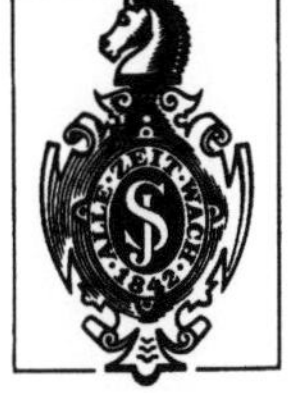

W. H. Lang · F. Muchel

ZEISS Microscopes for Microsurgery

With a Foreword by H. L. Wullstein

With 143 Figures and 5 Nomograms

Springer-Verlag Berlin Heidelberg New York 1981

Walter H. Lang
Dipl.-Phys. Dr. rer. nat.
Wissenschaftlicher Leiter der
Abteilung für Medizinische Geräte
Carl Zeiss, Oberkochen

Franz L. Muchel
Dipl.-Phys.
Leiter der
Mathematischen Abteilung für
Mikroskopie und Medizinische Geräte
Carl Zeiss, Oberkochen

ISBN-13:978-3-642-81646-8   e-ISBN-13:978-3-642-81644-4
DOI: 10.1007/978-3-642-81644-4

Library of Congress Cataloging in Publication Data

Lang, Walter H. 1931–.
ZEISS microscopes for microsurgery.
Bibliography: p. Includes index. 1. Microsurgery-Instruments.
2. Microscope and microscopy. I. Muchel, Franz L., 1932–.
II. Title. [DNLM: 1. Microsurgery-Instrumentation.
WO 162 L271z] RD33.6L36 617'.05 81-8787 AACR2

2061/3020/543210

Foreword in retrospect of a surgeon

Prof. Dr. med. Horst Ludwig Wullstein
Emeritus Director of the ENT Clinic of Würzburg University

Microsurgery, a hitherto inaccessible "new dimension in surgery", inaugurated a new era of surgical knowledge and treatment similar to the radical change brought about by antisepsis, asepsis and anaesthesia. Natural science and technology had frequently offered the conditions for a decisive step forward in medical science, enabling theoretical and clinical medicine to solve problems on which these had concentrated their efforts more or less extensively.

In two surgical disciplines in particular better vision was needed for further refinement than was obtainable with magnifying spectacles. In the years of complete destruction after World War II, one of the most miserable and helpless periods of Germany's intellectual and economic life, Zeiss scientists – above all Dr. H. Littmann – though starting virtually from scratch, offered in 1953 an operation microscope with all the characteristic features required by the profession. This instrument was so readily adaptable to all future developments that it scored great worldwide success. It is due to this early model that the terms operation microscope and Zeiss microscope have become almost synonymous, because all future designs were based on the principle of this very first instrument.

After 30 years of designing operation microscopes the Zeiss scientists Dr. W. H. Lang and Dipl.-Phys. Franz Muchel have now written a monograph on the design and equipment of this "tool" for a new kind of surgery. The authors asked me for a foreword from the point of view of a surgeon, because one of the first, perhaps even the first operation microscope supplied for constant use was set up in my operation room. I feel very much honored by the authors' request with which I am glad to comply.

To see more has always been an ardent desire of physicians. In the first half of the 19th century the mirror had become a most valuable aid used on the one hand for observation of the mirror image in dentistry and later adopted in other areas so far inaccessible to direct observation such as larynx and nasopharynx, and on the other hand particularly for illumination (also with a prism, Helmholtz) in ophthalmology and otology. With respect to the chief sense functions vision and hearing, eye and ear, there was for different reasons a strong demand to see more details in areas which are anatomically suited for transillumination or illumination. As far as the eye is concerned these are the transparent, refractive surface media, while the corresponding areas of the ear lie in the inner ear, the deeply sunk organ of hearing. Owing to its functional connection with the infection-prone respiratory passages, the inner ear was the source of many serious and lethal diseases of the skull base. Meningitis, for instance, dreaded at all times, had its source mostly in an inflammation in the middle ear.

However, not inflammatory but other functional disturbances of hearing between middle and inner ear, above all otosclerosis as a prototype disease, had in 1921 induced Nylén, then Assistant Medical Director of the Stockholm University Ear Clinic, to use a monocular microscope for surgery. G. Holmgreen, Nylén's teacher, used a binocular microscope in 1922. Nylén occupied himself for years with the elaboration of the principles of the method. The first renowned surgeons who continued the surgical treatment of otosclerosis contented themselves with magnifying spectacles. The only exception was G. Shambaugh Jr. on whose initiative a handier microscope was developed in 1942. Illumination was realized by means of a prism arranged between the objectives. The single microscopes which gradually come to be built were bulky and immobile, with unsatisfactory working distances and illumination systems, etc. In 1948/49 I had built for my own use an easily movable instrument consisting of a $10\times$ Leitz magnifier mounted on the stand and swivel arm of a dental engine. It brought an immediate, vehement rush of people with defective hearing, and from 1949 to 1953 I carried out more than 1000 operations with this instrument. F. Zöllner had a similar model built by Messrs. Fischer.

After decades of attempts made by a few surgeons the Zeiss microscope marked the turn of a new era. Apart from the superior optical quality, the Zeiss engineers had provided all necessary facilities and capabilities such as excellent coaxial illumination, changeable high-power stereo observation, focusing, easy magnification change at one and the same working distance, a stable, mobile stand, a strong smoothly movable carrier arm and a movable microscope body. The manufacturer has continually improved the microscope and extended its application to many different surgical disciplines and every conceivable problem in operation rooms, to training and instruction, and to the different kinds of documentation and image transmission. This treatise describes the great efforts Zeiss scientists and engineers undertook in creating the essential prerequisites for modern surgery. No surgeon or diagnostician will be able to realize and acknowledge the enormous efforts made on his behalf unless he has read this monograph.

It is easily understood in view of the worldwide dissemination of the operation microscope that its success began with the solution to most intricate surgical problems in the deep and narrow cavities of the lateral skull base, the middle ear in the immediate vicinity of such delicate structures as the inner ear with its functions, the meninx of two cranial fossae, the large veins and the cerebral artery within the petrosal bone, and the facial nerve. Surgery of the temporal bone thus became the first example of peripheral nerve microsurgery.

Nylén's first microscope had virtually no working distance and did not allow continuous working. The working distance of our "self-made" instruments was long enough for long-term uninterrupted surgical treatment under stringent aseptic conditions, but only at one magnification, which means one working distance anyhow. The Zeiss microscope by Dr. H. Littmann was the first to offer sharp images at every magnification and working distance, a prerequisite hardly appreciated by modern surgeons especially when they use zoom systems.

A microscope's working distance must fulfill two requirements: it must allow the manipulation of instruments, on the one hand adapted to the surgeon's eyes when he is in relaxed, upright position yet not too long, so that the position of the arms is correct and natural, on the other hand long enough for the introduction of long instruments in narrow and deep operating channels. Long instruments are required particularly at high magnifications, and their manipulation must be safe and smooth. Short-angled finger-tip instruments are not suitable. Special instruments had to be developed which could be moved without effort in all directions. In the depth of the temporal bone, the first important field of surgery, the extremely hard bone of the eburnated inner ear capsule and the open membranes of the sense organ are directly adjacent to one another within the operating field. This bone had to therefore be thinned down (1/10 mm was achieved, repeatedly checked with a measuring eyepiece) so that it could be cut even with an extremely fine sickel knife. For such special tasks as clockwise and counterclockwise grinding along sense organs and vascular walls, I introduced the diamond ball in bone surgery. Every surgical discipline had requirements of its own, be it an exactly and rigidly fixed microscope body in ophthalmosurgery, be it a microscope body of utmost mobility in cerebral surgery (Yaşargil) for which point haemostasis by monopolar coagulation was of great help.

Some thousand operation microscopes were in use in otology before the instrument was adopted in other disciplines, primarily a result of verbal information. Longer working distances allowed in ENT diagnosis and endolaryngeal surgery as well as endonasal and ethmoidal surgery of the hypophysis. Interest though belated then spread to ophthalmosurgery. In my opinion this is due to the fact that in spite of all topographical difficulties absolute immobility in the area of the skull base has decisive advantages the easily movable eyeball lacks. For surgical treatment under an operation microscope instead of observation alone, every muscular activity of the eyeball must be eliminated, which requires uniform anaesthesia and muscle relaxation. After ophthalmology peripheral nerve surgery adopted the operation microscope, followed by vascular surgery (symposia 1971 in Vienna and 1973 in Lisbon), which also promoted the development of operating techniques for surgical treatment of the basis encephali. While in the above-mentioned disciplines surgical treatment under the microscope is primarily a one-man job, the development of the diploscope made the help of an assistant possible in hand surgery. Last but not least microsurgery was adopted in gynaecology (fallopian tube) and urology (ureter and vesicle wall). Large skin grafts with pedicle, which replaced the difficult, imperiled pediculated flap closures then marked a radical change in plastic surgery which in the narrow sense of the word is surface surgery.

Summarizing the above one can say that the reconstruction of arteries, veins, nerves and tendines together with tissue biology have ultimately led to the astounding results of traumatology and traumatosurgery in re-implanting partly or completely cut-off limbs in functional condition. The operation microscope has become an indispensable tool in all fields of surgery.

To be a good microsurgeon is considered an honor nowadays, while in its early days microsurgery was only smiled at by those concerned with general surgery. Today future microsurgeons are given every assistance and have specimens of corpses and carcasses at their disposal for training purposes.

Why is microsurgery much more arduous than macrosurgery? Well, a microsurgical operation may last for hours, surgical treatment of extended glomus tumors of the viscerocranium of the temporal bone, for instance. I think the reasons are the following:

1. A microsurgeon works generally without or almost without assistance (exceptions are plastic, hand and re-implantation surgery). A microsurgeon does not interrupt surgical treatment if an assistant makes a ligature, for instance, he does not even lift his head when he receives another instrument, but works without interruption and relaxation.

2. When an instrument appears in the microscope's field of view the extensive motion of the hand must be changed to an optically translated motion within a narrow area. The eye is capable of guiding the hand laterally at $10\times$ or $25\times$ magnification, even without armrests, provided the illumination is satisfactory. Microsurgery is possible only under threedimensional observation, and manipulations become difficult at high magnifications because of the lack of depth of focus. The constant change from observation to treatment and vice versa will never be a mere reflex or a process that can be learned by training but must be subcortically controlled.

3. The unnatural immobility of the eyes which are bound to the eyepieces is most exacting during hours and hours of surgical treatment. Even during extended microscopic observations a microscopist will raise his head now and then, to exchange a specimen, for instance, and will feel relieved. A microsurgeon can never relax but works without interval, and the unnatural immobility of the eyeballs which are normally incessantly moving is most arduous. That's why microsurgery is much more strenuous than macrosurgery, and why quite a few surgeons do not spend enough time on the necessary training, especially if they do not have good threedimensional visual capacity.

Sophisticated techniques, new problems and methods of surgical treatment have evolved since 1953 Zeiss scientists and engineers made available to the profession the first yet perfect tool for surgery under the microscope. The operation microscope has radically changed the style of surgical treatment and opened in medicine a "new dimension of surgery".

Würzburg, March 1981

Preface

This book has been conceived as a reference for all those who want to deepen their knowledge of technical details, design concept and interaction of the individual modules of Zeiss operation microscopes. The subjects of the book are classified in accordance with our intention.
Special emphasis has been placed on practical hints for the user of operation microscopes to avoid operating errors. Parameters which are of paramount importance for surgeon and assistant such as PD and diopter setting are therefore described in detail. The effects of wrong adjustments are indicated. The above statements also apply to the ample selection of accessories for Zeiss operation microscopes. That is why much attention has been given to the accessories for co-observation and documentation.
The most frequently used formulae are listed in the last chapter of the book, supplemented by nomograms which allow the reader to determine the most important data of a specific piece of microscope equipment without calculation.
Our thanks are due to all those who assisted in preparing the manuscript, drawings and photographs, to Mrs. Ursula Gabler for making the English translation and Miss Helen Robertson for editing it, and last but not least to the Springer-Verlag for the most careful, qualified and excellent production of the book.

Oberkochen, March 1981   Walter H. Lang   Franz Muchel

Table of contents

1 The technical principle of operation microscopes

1.1 Minimum demands on magnifying systems: prism loupes

An operation microscope is a special magnifying system. In a narrower sense spectacles of different technical design and 2× to 8× magnification are known as visual aids. Assuming that an operation field is adequately illuminated by means other than the visual aid itself, the minimum demands are as follows.

a) A visual aid must produce an *enlarged* image of the operating field for better visibility of minute features; only then is the transition from normal to microsurgery possible.

b) The enlarged image of the operating field must be *upright* and *unreversed* to relieve the surgeon of reorientation in the use of the microinstruments, and allow him to concentrate fully on the microsurgical procedure in progress.

c) An image corresponding to the specifications of a) and b) must be *three-dimensional* for satisfactory depth perception in the operating field, which means that a stereoscopic image should be produced of operating field and microinstruments.

d) To introduce microinstruments into the field of view and use them conveniently a certain distance, the so-called *working distance* is necessary between the front surface of the low vision aid and the operating field, which from experience should be at least 150 mm.

e) Last but not least the *color* of the operating field must be *faithfully* reproduced for precise detail recognition.

These minimum requirements are fulfilled not only by operation microscopes but also by Zeiss prism loupes. These systems use small binoculars of the Kepler telescope design, and with clip-on lenses of short focal length meet all demands specified under a) through e) above. The systems are "lightweights".

Fig. 1 shows schematically the design of the Zeiss mini binoculars with direct-vision prism. Their principal element is a Pechan prism which consists of two combined glass prisms arranged between objective and eyepiece of the Kepler telescope. This prism erects and reverses the inverted and reversed image of the astronomical telescope. For near vision, that is on the prism magnifying spectacles, a lens of suitable focal length is clipped onto the objective.

Different prism magnifying spectacles are shown in Figs. 2 to 4. The simplest model is spectacles as fixture of a modified small binocular (Fig. 2). For correction of ametropia such spectacles must be fitted by an optician (Fig. 3) The modified binoculars

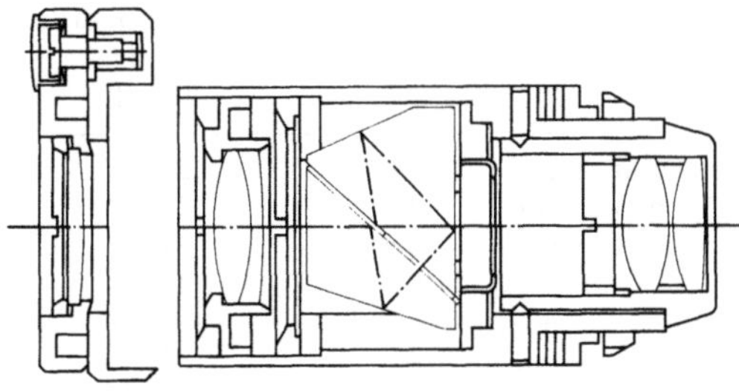

Fig. 1. Design principle of Zeiss mini binoculars from which the Zeiss magnifying spectacles are derived. Prism magnifying system (3.8 × magnification).

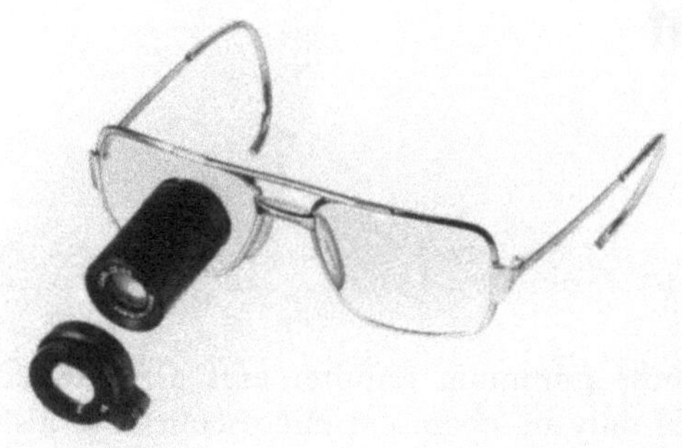

Fig. 2. Simplest model of prism magnifying spectacles.

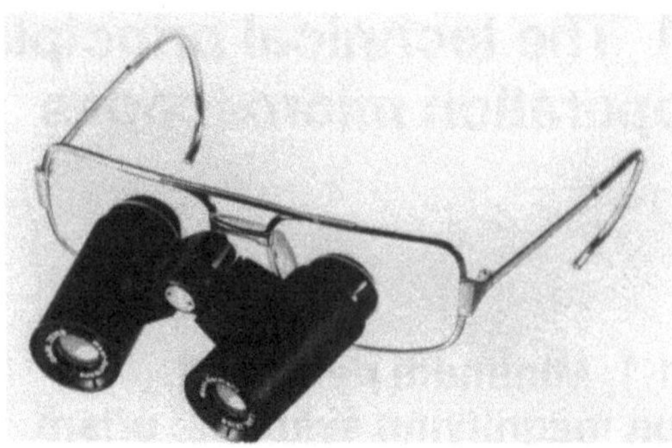

Fig. 3. Prism magnifying spectacles with correction lenses

can be mounted on a headband (Fig. 4) which also accepts illumination equipment for the operating field.

Table 1 lists the Zeiss prism magnifying spectacles with magnifications ranging from 3× to 8×. The distance between eye and operating field depends on the desired magnification, and ranges from 195 mm to 315 mm. The working distance can be roughly determined by subtracting the length of the binoculars from this distance; depending on the degree of ametropia the value lies between 48.5 and 60.5 mm. (For an exact calculation of the working distance the distance between spectacle lens and vertex of the cornea must also be considered.)

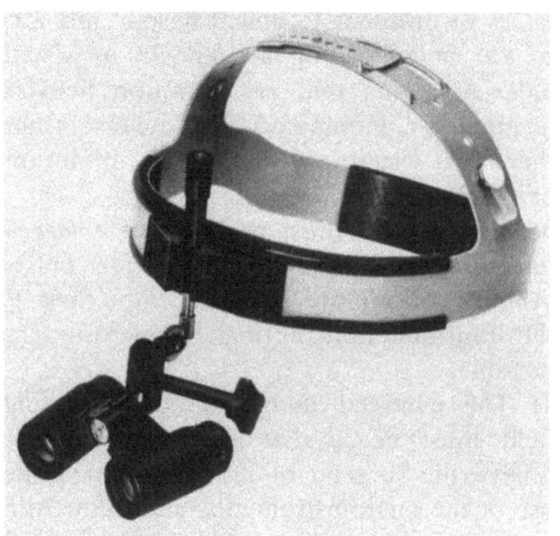

Fig. 4. Prism headband magnifiers

Table 1. Technical data of Zeiss prism loupes

	Magnification	Distance eye to operating field [mm]	Length [mm]	Field-of-view dia. [mm]	Weight [g]
Binocularsystem in frame *without* corrective lenses	4×	310	from 48.5 to	58	approx. 97
	5×	270	59.5 acc. to	48	
	6×	240	ametropia	39	
	8×	200		30	
Binocularsystem in frame *with* corrective lenses	3×	315	49.5 to 60.5	62	approx 110 with holder without frame
	4×	270		43	
	5×	240		35	
	6×	220		30	
	8×	195		22	

In general surgery and in microsurgery in particular the practical use of prism loupes or similar systems aids is limited by a maximum useful magnification. Magnifying spectacles follow every movement of the head. This blurs the image they produce of an object structure, because the object features in the field of view change more or less rapidly. This is the more disturbing the faster the movement of the head. These properties exclude magnifying spectacles from prolonged use in microsurgery, and create a demand for visual aids without such drawbacks. Further, new features were required of magnifying visual aids for microsurgery, which will be discussed later. From these evolved the operation microscope which has become an indispensable tool in modern microsurgery.

1.2 Additional demands on magnifying systems: operation microscopes

The sequence in which these demands are mentioned below is no measure of their importance. The requirements vary considerably from one application or medical discipline to the other. This list includes only the most important, constantly recurring demands and does not lay claim to completeness. The following statements supplement paras. a) to e) of section 1.1.

f) As the sophistication of microsurgical techniques and instruments constantly increased, higher magnifications (2 to 40×) of the operating field and the microinstruments introduced became necessary. Magnifications up to 60× have been used in exceptional cases. This is a practical upper limit of useful magnification which is contested for operation microscopes.

g) Microsurgical procedures generally require more than just one magnification, which necessitates a magnification changer for a given magnification range without modification of the operation microscope itself.

h) In microsurgery the optimum working distance varies from 150 mm to 400 mm depending on the application. In otorhinolaryngology, for instance, an operation microscope must be adjustable to 200 mm working distance for surgery of the middle ear, or to 400 mm for laryngology, without time-consuming modifications of the microscope.

i) The image quality is of minor importance at low magnifications, and was therefore not mentioned among the minimum requirements; moreover high image quality is characteristic of modern optical systems. But the higher the magnification the more important the image quality. The image in an operation microscope must be perfectly flat, with spherical, astigmatic and chromatic aberrations below the limit of perception.

j) Adequate image quality also means adequate resolving power. Especially at high magnifications an operation microscope's resolving power must be near the theoretically feasible value. Just how important the demands i) and j) are, is revealed when an operation microscope is used at high magnifications for hours without interruption as, for instance, in neurosurgery for an intercranial operation.

k) As mentioned under c), magnifying visual aids must produce a three-dimensional image of the operating field also at low magnifications. This applies, of course, also to operation microscopes or, more precisely, at a high magnification and a long working distance an operation microscope must produce a stereoscopic impression of an object in the operating field that satisfies the demands of microsurgical procedures.

l) When the magnification increases at a given working distance, the size of the area, in which object structures are clearly visible in the microscope's viewing direction decreases. Outside this so-called depth-of-focus range, which has no sharply defined boundaries, objects appear blurred and are of low contrast. A wide depth-of-focus range is necessary; otherwise the microscope must constantly be re-focused if the depth extension of objects varies (intervertebral disks, for instance).

m) At low magnifications the illumination of the operating field is not critical, because operating lamps provide adequate illumination. At high magnifications, however, special light sources are needed, which should preferably be connected with the operation microscope. Coaxial illumination systems which illuminate the operating field through the microscope during observation are a pre-condition for microsurgery in or through narrow body cavities (vitreous surgery).

n) Depending on the discipline, the surgical technique, and the type of operation microscope, the instrument must frequently be re-adjusted and the magnification changed. The whole instrument or at least its critical parts must therefore be sterile. (This does not apply if a microscope is completely covered by sterile cloths or plastic covers, or if all adjusting actions are motorized).

o) An operation microscope and its accessories must be absolutely reliable, and always ready in case of emergencies, even after improper use or extended periods of nonuse. Especially during an operation the microscope as a whole and all its parts must always function properly and no breakdowns are permissible. In instruments with integral illumination system, the light sources are the parts most susceptible to breakdowns. Before the start of a critical operation provision should therefore be made for makeshift continuation until, for instance, a defective light source can be replaced.

p) Varying but always stringent safety reg-

ulations for operating theaters are in force in different countries, which must be strictly followed. This applies in particular to electrical safety regulations and provisions for explosion hazards. It is absolutely necessary to obtain a design registration of microscope type and accessories in countries with stringent safety regulations.

q) In some medical disciplines an assistant is needed not only for training and instruction but also for performing microsurgery. The assistant uses a second operation microscope which must offer the same view of the operating field as the surgeon's. In some disciplines (hand surgery) two assistant's microscopes are necessary.

r) Documentation facilities are indispensable in research and development and for training and instruction; they must be compatible with every operation microscope.

s) The instrument nurse's work can be considerably facilitated by co-observation facilities on the operation microscope, which are, of course, also of great importance for training and instruction.

t) An operation microscope and fitted accessories must be easy to operate, especially if a microscope has to be adjusted to different viewing directions during surgery (inner ear surgery). For these surgical procedures microscope and accessories must be well balanced by counterweights.

u) In all fields of microsurgery small dimensions of the microscope guarantee a better survey of the area surrounding of the operating field.

v) Only a lightweight microscope can be adjusted without effort.

w) Safe and stable mounting of the microscope on special arms and couplings for the various fields of microsurgery is of particular importance at high microscope magnifications.

x) These demands on an operation microscope are so complex that a modular system is the only economically feasible solution.

It must be possible to attach and exchange compatible modules without the need of tools.

y) It must be possible to attach special equipment such as an electronic flash or the motorized operation slit lamp to every old or new operation microscope model.

z) Last but not least, the maintenance of an operation microscope should not present any difficulties even to inexperienced personnel.

1.3 Diagrams illustrating the design principle of Zeiss operation microscopes

The design of the simplest Zeiss operation microscope [2] is based on a suggestion by Barraquer (Fig. 5). The operating field should lie in the microscope's focal plane, here situated in the object focal plane of

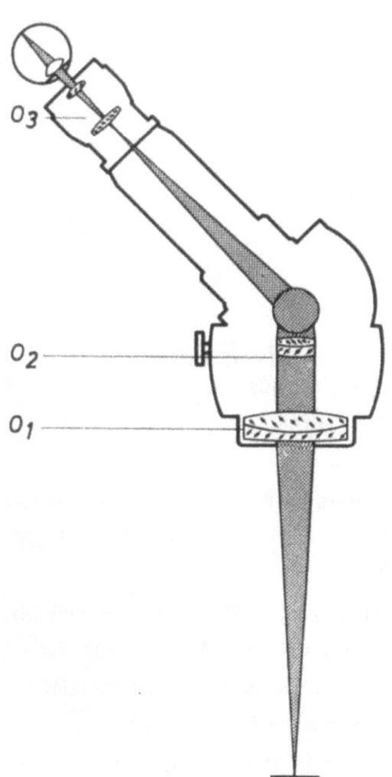

Fig. 5. Design principle of an operation microscope without magnification changer. O_1 primary objective; O_2 tube lens; O_3 eyepiece.

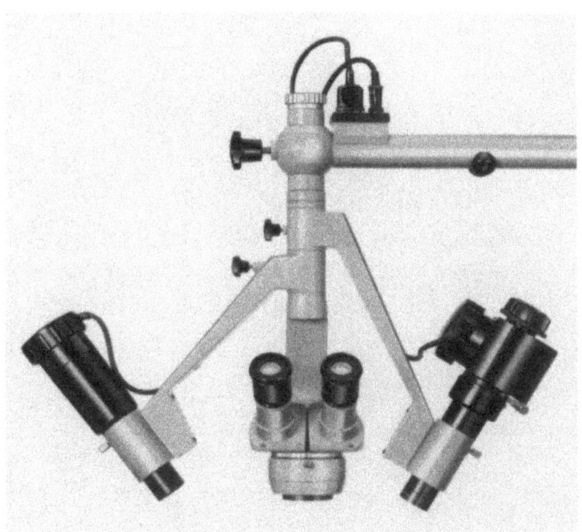

Fig. 6. Operation microscope Opmi 3 without magnification changer.

the microscope objective; the image of the operating field is produced at infinity. This idea is also called "parallel beam path" above the objective. For a finite image or, more exactly, an image at a given site in an operation microscope, a convergent optical system of short focal length (125 or 160 mm) must be provided in the microscope's binocular tube. An image of the operating field is then produced in the so-called eyepiece plane. This image is viewed through eyepieces and, enlarged for instance, $10\times$, $12.5\times$ or $16\times$. Fig. 6 shows this microscope type. As it has no integral illumination system, a homogeneous and a slit illuminator are mounted on the microscope side. Because of the simplicity of the design and the ease of operation, the operation microscope after Barraquer has become a standard instrument in ophthalmic microsurgery.

The following three features of this microscope type deserve special mention [9 d]. The first is the microscope objective which is used like a magnifier: the objective produces at infinity an image of the object field which lies in its front focal plane. Objectives of different focal length and different working distance can therefore be

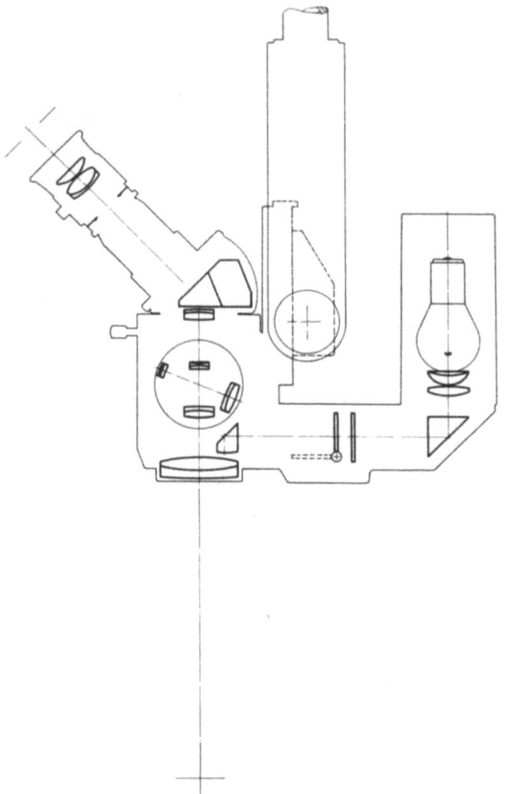

Fig. 7. Design principle of an operation microscope with 5-stage magnification changer (Opmi 1).

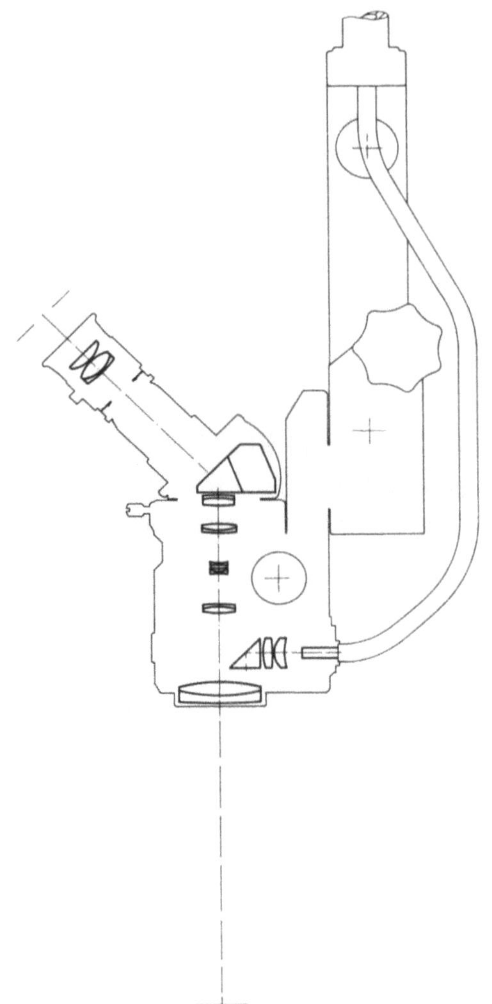

Fig. 9. Design principle of an operation microscope with zoom system and integral fiber-optics illumination.

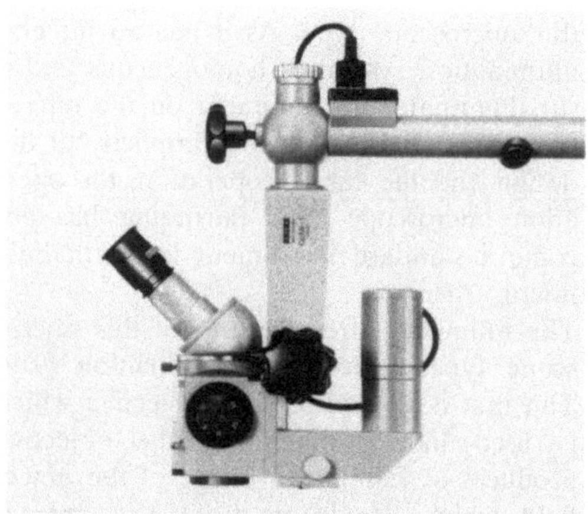

Fig. 8. Operation microscope built according to the design principle shown in Fig. 7.

used (homogeneous and slit illuminator must, of course, be adjusted to the objective focal length).

The second feature is the parallel beam path between objective and binocular tube, that is inside the microscope, which allows provision of a magnification changer in the microscope body and/or a beam splitter to utilize part of the reflected light for co-observation or documentation (details see Chapter 6).

The third feature is a finite image produced in the binocular tube after the parallel beam path from the microscope body is accepted at the entrance of the binocular tube. In practice different binocular tubes can thus be used with different focal lengths of the convergent optical system. Binocular tubes of 125 mm and 160 mm focal length are the most frequently used.

This design principle applies to all Zeiss microscopes and is a pre-condition for the modular design of an operation microscope.

Figs. 7 and 8 show design principle and final version of a more sophisticated operation microscope [9a, 9b] with integral illumination system and 5-stage magnification changer (details see description of the individual modules). Figs. 9 and 10 show one of the latest operation microscopes [9c] with integral fiber-optics illumination and zoom magnification systems. The individual modules of the microscope and its accessories are described in the following chapter.

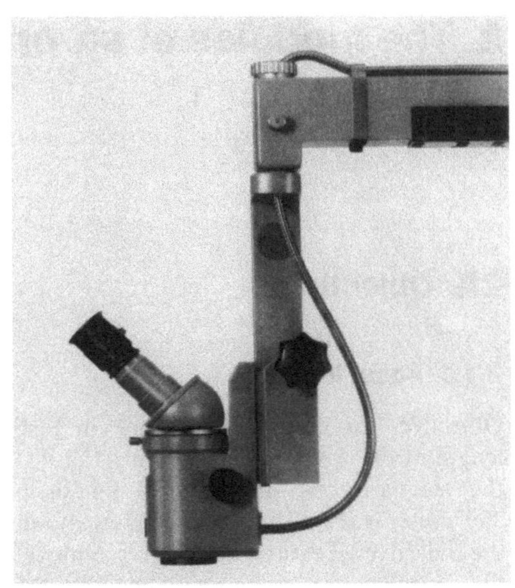

Fig. 10. Operation microscope Opmi 6 F built according to the design principle shown in Fig. 9.

2 The modules of an operation microscope

2.1 Objectives

2.1.1 Focal length

Objectives for microsurgery come in focal lengths from 150 mm to 400 mm (Fig. 11); the standard one has a focal length of 200 mm (Fig. 12). Thanks to a screw mount the objectives are easily attached or removed for exchange or cleaning. The objective

2.1.2 Working distance

The *working distance a* of an operation microscope is by definition equal to the distance between the front lens vertex and the object plane, that is the "plane" of the operating field. The working distance is approximately (less than 5% deviation) equal to the focal length of the objective. The longer the focal length the better the approximation.

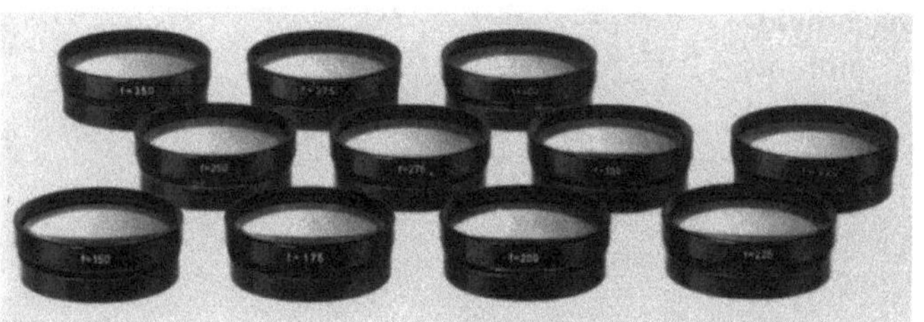

Fig. 11. Objectives for microsurgery.

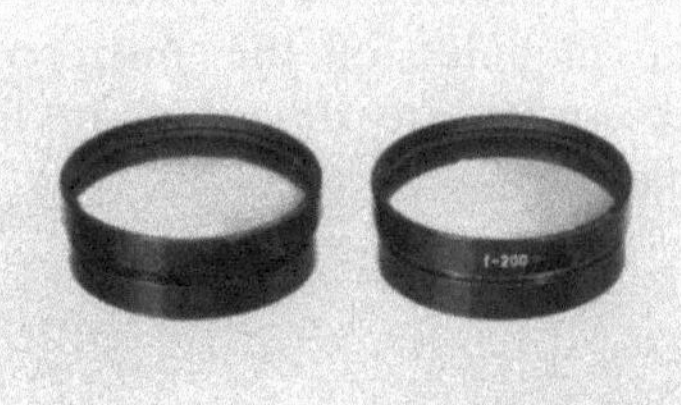

Fig. 12. Objective of 200 mm focal length.

mount is engraved with trademark, serial number and, for instance, $f = 200$, which indicates that this objective has a *focal length* of 200 mm.

The distance from the lens center to the focal plane, that is the plane of the operating field (see section 1.3) is the focal length of thin lenses (Fig. 13). Because of the required high image quality objectives of operation microscopes are thicker and consist of at least two cemented elements (Fig. 13). A principal plane, which for an objective of 200 mm focal length, for instance, lies 5.3 mm behind the front lens vertex is taken as origin for the calculation of the focal length of such cemented component lenses.

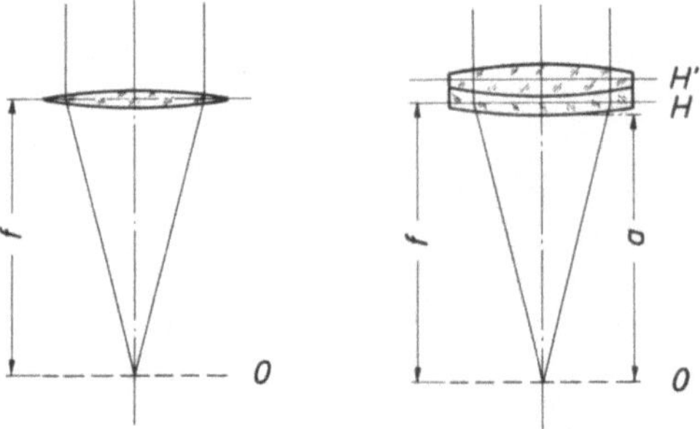

Fig. 13. The focal length f of a thin lens (left) is the distance from the lens center. The focal length f of the thick lenses in the objectives of operation microscopes is the distance from the front principal plane H. The focal plane O is identical with the object field (operating field). H' is the rear principal plane which is irrelevant in this connection. a is the working distance.

2.1.3 Image quality

Every optical system has unavoidable, more or less conspicuous optical deficiencies which impair the image quality. These aberrations are corrected when computing an optical system to minimize their influence. The quality of an optical system depends ultimately on the extent to which *all* potential image aberrations can be eliminated in the computation, design and finally series production of the system. Only optics of superior quality can be used in an operation microscope, and these optics are characterized by the *simultaneous* correction of *all* aberrations to such an extent that they are no longer perceptible. This requirement, which can be realized in practice, must be fulfilled not only by the microscope objective but by all other optical parts of an operation microscope as well. If optics of inferior quality are used, the one or the other aberration or even several at a time become noticeable and interfere with observation. This stresses the surgeon unnecessarily, especially when he works with the instrument for hours without interruption. Fatigue and lack of concentration are the result, diverting the surgeon from microsurgery proper.

Zeiss operation microscopes are time-tested modular systems, especially tailored to the needs of clinical surgery, which accept various accessories for assistants, co-observation and documentation. This is only possible in a system whose modules "fit" mechanically and optically. Besides, newly developed accessories must be adaptable to every operation microscope, be it new or 10 years old or more. This explains even to a technically less experienced person why every single module of an operation microscope must meet the highest quality standards.

Merely for the sake of completeness some image aberrations are listed below in an order which corresponds to the frequency with which they occur in operation microscopes and accessories of lesser quality.

a) **Distortion** is the most easily recognized aberration. Straight sides of a square bulge (barrel distortion) or are concave (pin-cushion distortion), especially towards the edge of the image.

b) **Chromatic aberration.** Color fringes along the defined boundaries of objects, which do not exist in the object and are considered artefacts.

c) **Spherical aberration.** Object features are blurred or minute details hardly visible; the image appears "foggy" or "turbid" which has, of course, direct influence on the microscope's resolving power. High magnifications cannot be used effectively.

d) **Field curvature.** If an image is not perfectly flat, a plane object appears curved. This aberration influences the visual impression of the axial extension of an object (in the microscope's viewing direction).

e) **Astigmatism.** Only an experienced user will notice it if the operating field is the object, but it is revealed by a test object consisting of concentric rings with radial spokes. With astigmatism rings and spokes are not in focus at the same time.

2.1.4 Anti-reflection coating

A look at an objective front surface against the light reveals a slight bluish tint which is due to an ultra-thin metal film. This anti-reflection coating suppresses disturbing reflections and stray light. Without it the microscopic image would be of low contrast. Contamination of the objective more or less counter acts the effect of the anti-reflection coating. It reduces the contrast and in extreme cases appears as a turbid veil over the microscopic image.

2.1.5 Image brightness

The working distance changes when exchanging an objective for another of different focal length. The brightness of the microscopic image changes as well, but this is not as obvious and easily understood, though it must be considered for photographic, cine and TV recording. The qualitative reason for the brightness change is easily explained, but one thing must be stated in advance.

When the objective of an operation microscope with 5-stage (Figs. 7 and 8) or zoom magnification system (Figs. 9 and 10) is unscrewed, two circular, de-centered openings of 16 mm diameter each (Fig. 14) are visible in the microscope body. The distance between the centers of the two openings is

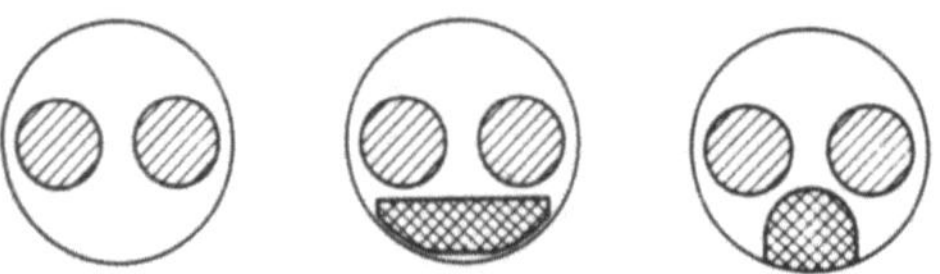

Fig. 14. Lower part of microscope body. Objective unscrewed (schematic drawing).

22 mm. These are the entrance openings of the observation beam path (hatched in Fig. 14). The cross-hatched areas are illuminating prisms, discussed in para. 3.3.1. Important for the observation and thus the brightness of the microscopic image are only the light beams which pass through the two openings. Fig. 15 shows schematically the side view of two objectives for operation microscopes of different focal length and different working distance. Starting from the center P of the operating field O the two hatched bundles pass through the objective and can reach the two entrance openings of the 5-stage magnification changer or zoom system. Assuming the intensity of the light coming from the object point P to be illustrated by the number of arrows, it is easily understood that – under otherwise equal conditions – the more light reaches the observation beam paths the shorter the working distance of the objective.

2.2 Binocular tubes

2.2.1 Straight tubes, inclined tubes

Binocular tubes for operation microscopes come in different types, primarily straight and inclined (Fig. 16). The two eyepiece tubes of the straight tubes are parallel with the microscope axis and offer a "straight" viewing direction on the operating field. The eyepiece tubes of inclined tubes form a 45°

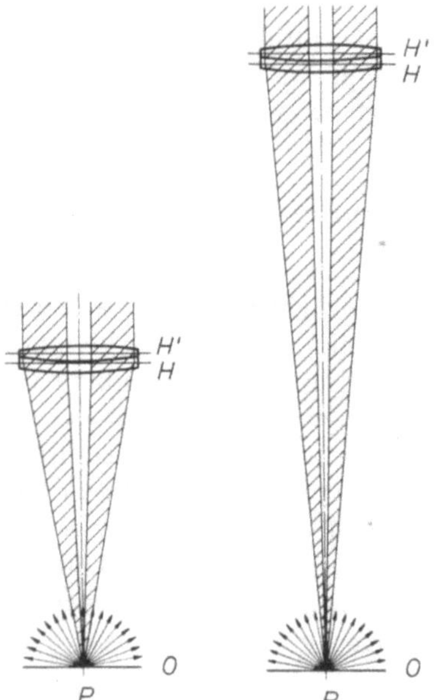

Fig. 15. The objective of short focal length takes up more light than that of long focal length. The brightness of the image with short focal-length objective is therefore greater.

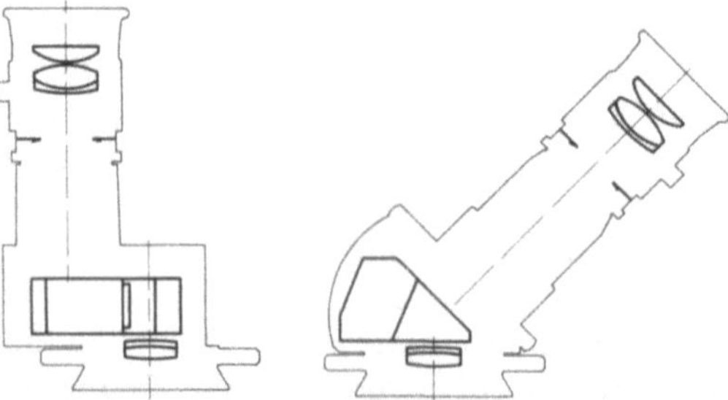

Fig. 16. Schematic representation of a straight tube (left) and an inclined tube (right).

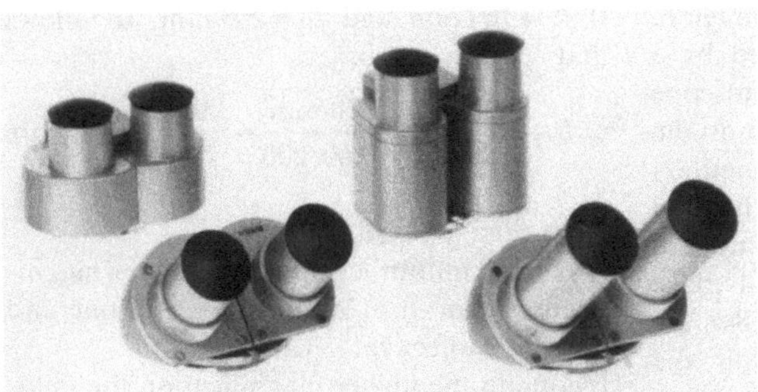

Fig. 17. Binocular tubes of 125 mm (left) and 160 mm (right) focal length.

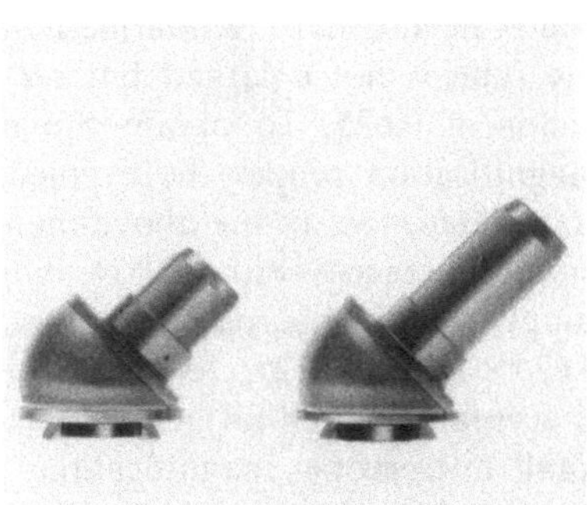

Fig. 18. Inclined tubes of 125 mm (left) and 160 mm (right) focal length.

angle with the microscope axis, and offer an "oblique" viewing direction on the operating field.

There are specific applications for both types. In ophthalmic microsurgery, for instance, the microscope axis is generally perpendicular to the eye or deviates only slightly from the vertical. Inclined tubes are therefore the choice for comfortable viewing. In otorhinolaryngology, for microsurgery of the larynx, for instance, a straight tube is needed for more convenient observation and manipulation of the microinstruments, while for a tympanoplasty an inclined tube is preferred. Both types may be applied in one and the same discipline, and the situation is similar in neurosurgery. Microscope body and binocular tube are provided with dovetails for easy exchange if an operation microscope is shared with other disciplines or equipped for different surgical techniques. The tube is secured with a knurled screw on the side of the tube facing the surgeon, Figs. 17 and 18 show different types of binocular tubes.

2.2.2 Focal lengths of binocular tubes

Apart from being straight or inclined, binocular tubes have different focal lengths. The term "focal length" used in connection with operation microscope's binocular tubes may be surprising, but remember sections 1.3 and 2.1: the objective of an operation microscope is used like a magnifier and therefore produces an image at infinity. Only a convergent optical system forms this image in the microscope or, more precisely, in the binocular tube. A so-called intermediate image is produced by the convergent system in the eyepiece plane, where it can be observed re-enlarged through the eyepiece. Different focal lengths of the convergent system lend themselves for microsurgery, 125 mm and 160 mm being the standard focal lengths of straight and inclined binocular tubes (Figs. 17 and 18). The focal length ($f = 125$ or $f = 160$) is imprinted on the tube. The two different focal lengths lead to:

a) **Different overall lengths** (Figs. 17 and 18), which permits the choice of a microscope which best suits the surgeon's height and offers the seated user the most comfortable working position.

b) **Different magnifications.** The effect of the objective that is used like a magnifier is reversed by the convergent system in the binocular tube. The magnification of the image in the intermediate plane of the binocular tube is calculated from the quotient of the tube focal length f_T and the objective focal length f_O. $f_T = 125$ mm and $f_O = 200$ mm result in a magnification in the intermediate image plane of the binocular tube of 125 mm/200 mm $= 0.625$. In this example the quotient f_T/f_O is smaller than 1, which means that the intermediate image in the tube is not enlarged but reduced by a factor of 0.625. To obtain the microscope magnification proper the eyepiece must be considered, too. In the above-mentioned example eyepieces with $12.5\times$ magnification supply a total microscope magnification of $0.625\times 12.5 = 7.8125$. As one decimal place is accurate enough for general use, 7.8 is the total microscope magnification. With the same objective $f_O = 200$ mm, but $f_T = 160$ mm the magnification in the intermediate image plane of the binocular tube will be 160 mm/200 mm = 0.8, and the total microscope magnification with $12.5\times$ eyepieces $0.8\times 12.5 = 10.0$. Simplified the task of objective and convergent system in the binocular tube can be expressed as follows: the "sole" purpose of the parameters objective focal length and binocular tube focal length is to establish a suitable distance between operation microscope and operating field, determine the overall length of the microscope, and produce in the eyepiece plane of the binocular tube an intermediate image without noticeable aberrations. Different binocular tube focal lengths also lead to

c) Different field-of-view diameters. This is the diameter of the circular operating field which is surveyed through the operation microscope. To illustrate the fact we use again a numerical example.

All eyepiece tubes of binocular tubes have at the site of the intermediate image an internal diameter of 20 mm. The field-of-view diameter of the operating field D_O can be calculated form this value, provided the magnification of the intermediate image in the eyepiece tubes of the binocular tube is known. According to b) it is 0.625 for $f_T = 125$ mm and $f_O = 200$ mm. It follows for the field-of-view diameter D_O of the operating field that

$$D_O = \frac{20 \text{ mm}}{f_T/f_O} = \frac{20 \text{ mm}}{125/200} = \frac{20 \text{ mm}}{0.625} = 32 \text{ mm}.$$

If $f_T = 160$ mm and $f_O = 200$ mm, it follows that

$$D_O = \frac{20 \text{ mm}}{f_T/f_O} = \frac{20 \text{ mm}}{160/200} = \frac{20 \text{ mm}}{0.8} = 25 \text{ mm}.$$

According to these examples
I) the 160 mm tube supplies a higher magnification than the 125 mm tube with one and the same objective;
II) due to the higher magnification the field-of-view diameter is smaller with the 160 mm than with the 125 mm tube.
These facts and the geometrical dimensions of the tubes must be considered for the choice of the binocular tube focal length in each individual case.

d) Image brightness. Another consequence of different binocular tube (and microscope objective) focal lengths is to mention: The higher the magnification the lower the brightness of the microscopic image, a fact which is of importance for the choice of modules and accessories for co-observation and documentation.

2.2.3 Interpupillary distance *(PD)*

a) *PD* **adjustment.** According to para. 2.1.5 the center distance of step or zoom magnification systems is always 22 mm (details see section 2.4). All binocular tubes must therefore have two entrance openings, each with a diameter of 16 mm, and a distance between the two centers of 22 mm. The surgeon's interpupillary distance (that is, the distance between the pupil centers of the two eyes) lies between 48 and 76 mm. These two, the fixed center distance of 22 mm and the surgeon's *PD* must be adapted. Technically this is achieved by a prism in each of the two beam paths, which causes a parallel shift of the observation axes. The binocular tubes must be so designed that both eyepiece tubes can be turned around an axis parallel to the axes of the eyepiece tubes. The range of this motion covers *PD*s from 48 mm to 76 mm.

With the latest binocular tubes the adjusted *PD* is indicated on a scale by an index line (Fig. 19). If the surgeon's *PD* is known an assistant can set it when preparing the microscope for operation. Otherwise it is determined as follows: set both eyepiece tubes to maximum *PD,* then turn them uniformly towards smaller values while looking through the binocular tube (with eyepieces). The

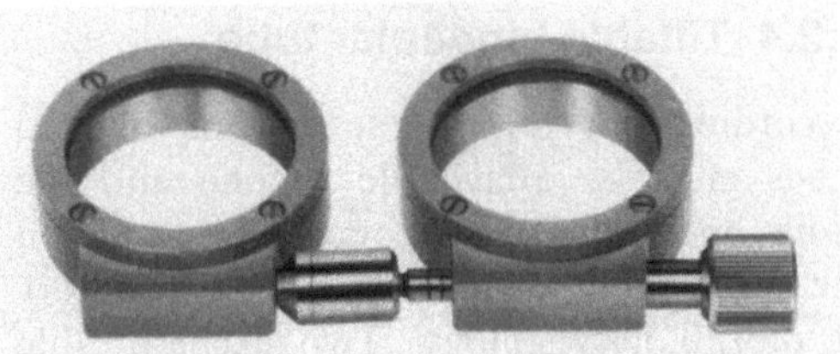

Fig. 20. PD adjuster for inclined tubes, also suitable for subsequent fitting.

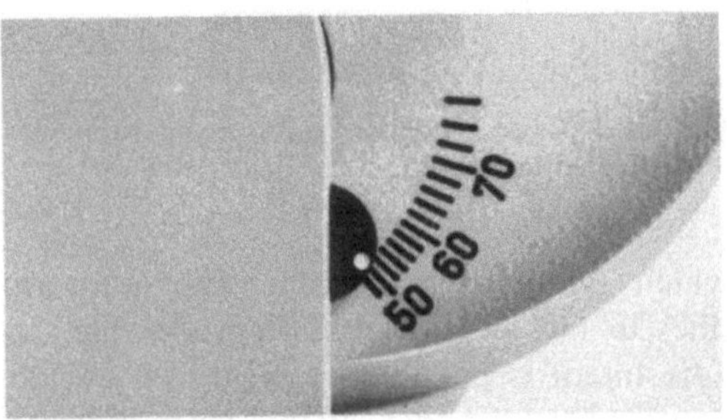

Fig. 19. Interpupillary distance (*PD*), scale with index line on the binocular tube.

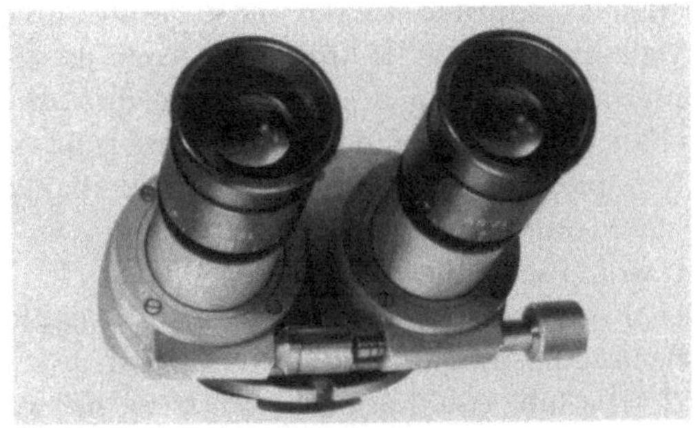

Fig. 21. *PD* adjuster mounted on inclined tube.

operating field can be seen with one eye only as long as the *PD* is much higher than the value to be found. Two images appear as the correct *PD* value is approached. The distance between the two images must be reduced until they coincide. The value thus achieved can be read off a scale; it is the surgeon's *PD*.

Exact *PD* adjustment is a pre-condition for stereoscopic vision. Even minor deviations from optimum adjustment impair the fusion of the two images into one three-dimensional image, or make it impossible. Correct *PD* adjustment is therefore necessary *before* starting to work with an operation microscope (more information see section 2.3).

b) *PD* adjuster. A surgeon may touch the binocular tube when changing the microscope's viewing direction during a surgical procedure, and he can do so without danger of unsterility if the binocular tube is covered by sterilizable rubber caps (see chapter 7). To avoid at the same time disadjustment of

the *PD* setting the motion around the folding axis of the binocular tube must be stiff so that an effort must be made to set the *PD*. This may be annoying if surgeon and assistant change places during an operation and the *PD* has to be re-set. It is difficult to combine this necessarily stiff motion which needs force to adjust it with the smoothness required for manipulation of the micro-instruments in a limited operating field.

The problem is solved by the *PD* adjuster for inclined tubes (Fig. 20). It can be subsequently fitted to existing binocular inclined tubes (Fig. 21) and has the following major advantages:

I) It can be operated without effort.

II) It can be operated with one hand (normal *PD* adjustment requires both hands because the motion is stiff).

III) A sterilizable cap is available for the knob.

IV) Disadjustment is impossible due to a self-locking mechanism of the *PD* adjuster.

2.2.4 Tiltable binocular tube

According to para. 2.2.1 straight or inclined tubes must be attachable to one and the same operation microscope, depending on the application, for instance, in neurosurgery or otorhinolaryngology. Two exchangeable binocular tubes must be available.

Straight and inclined tubes have fixed viewing angles, which has unpleasant consequences: before an operation the surgeon's chair is adjusted to the most comfortable viewing position. If the microscope is repositioned during a surgical procedure the chair often is not, and conditions are similarly unpleasant if surgeon and assistant change places during an operation.

It would solve the problem

I) if one and the same binocular tube could be used in straight or inclined position;

II) if a tube could not only be set to the two extreme positions (straight or inclined) but also to any position in between;

III) if such a universal tube were equipped with a *PD* adjuster according to para. 2.2.3b.

The tiltable binocular tube (Fig. 22) fulfills all three requirements. The viewing tubes can be angulated through 60° and locked in any position between straight and inclined (Fig. 23). The adjusted tilt is indicated on a scale. The tilting mechanism is self-locking

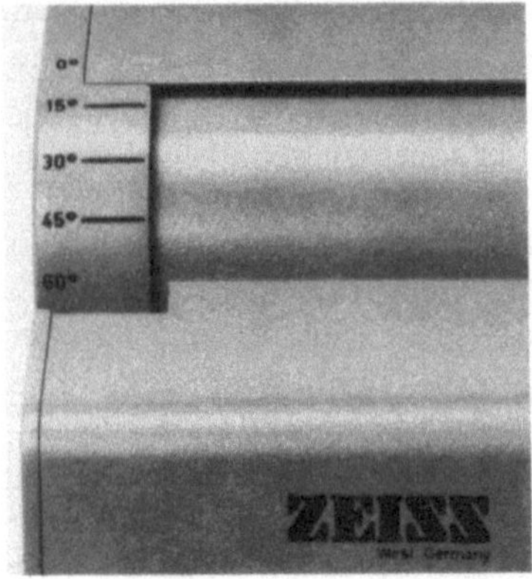

Fig. 23. Tiltable binocular tube. Scale for viewing-angle adjustment.

which avoids disadjustment. The same applies to the *PD* adjuster. Reproducible *PD* adjustment is possible by means of a scale. Sterilizable caps are available for both items. For the 60° tiltable binocular tube special screw-mount eyepieces have been developed which cannot be pulled out of the correct position by mistake as normal eyepieces can (see also section 2.3). The eyepieces accept micrometer disks. The tiltable binocular tube has a focal length of 160 mm. The design does not allow shorter focal lengths, e.g. 125 mm.

The tiltable binocular tube has the further major advantage that it reduces the effective overall length of the operation microscope, a point which is discussed in detail later.

The tiltable binocular tube is attachable to all current and earlier models of Zeiss operation microscopes.

2.3 Eyepieces

2.3.1 General functions

The microscope objective and the convergent system in the binocular tube produce an intermediate image in the intermediate image plane of the binocular tube (see also section 1.3). The intermediate image of the

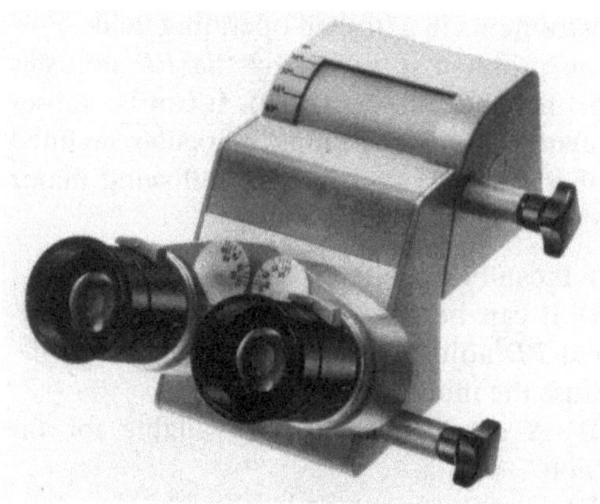

Fig. 22. Tiltable binocular tube.

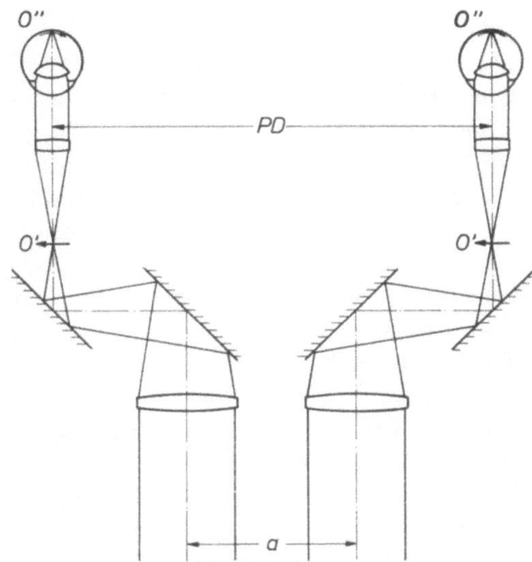

Fig. 24. The interrelationship of binocular tube and eyepiece (schematic). O' intermediate image plane; O'' image on the retina; PD interpupilary distance.

operating field is generally reduced not enlarged. The enlargement is done by the eyepieces, using a pair of them like a magnifier. It is not necessary to constantly readjust the eyepieces to the intermediate image, because

I) the intermediate image in the operation microscope produced by objective and binocular tube is always situated in the intermediate image plane of the two eyepiece tubes (Fig. 24);

The primary task of the eyepieces is to enlarge the intermediate image produced in the binocular tubes to the desired value.

II) an eyepiece pair of given magnification has a definite, known focal length. If the eyepieces are pushed in the eyepiece tubes *as far as they will go,* the correct distance between eyepieces and intermediate image is automatically established. In other words: if the eyepieces are in this prescribed position, the intermediate image to be enlarged lies in the front focal plane of the eyepieces;

III) an annular stop in the eyepiece limits the field of view and is arranged so as to coincide with the intermediate image plane of the eyepiece tube.

With a given working distance of the objective and a given focal length of the binocular tube (without consideration of the magnification changer) different magnifications are only obtainable by eyepieces of different focal length (Fig. 25).

2.3.2 Individual functions

a) Microscope magnification and field-of-view diameter. Trademark and magnification are engraved on every eyepiece. Eyepieces are available of the suitable graded magnifications $10\times$, $12.5\times$, $16\times$, $20\times$ (Fig. 25), i.e. the magnification rises by a factor of 1.25. The choice of the eyepiece depends on the desired and/or necessary total microscope magnification. In operation microscopes without magnification changer the total magnification depends on the focal length of the microscope objective f_O, the focal length of the binocular tube f_T, and the eyepiece magnification V_E. The total magnification of an operation microscope *without* magnifi-

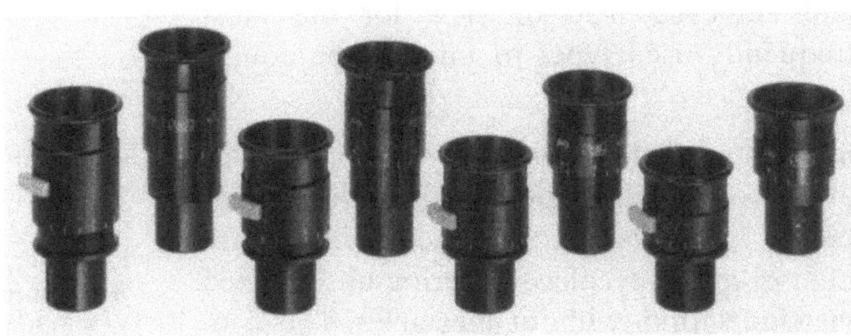

Fig. 25. Eyepieces for $10\times$, $12.5\times$, $16\times$ and $20\times$ magnification.

cation changer is calculated with the formula

$$\frac{f_{\mathrm{T}}}{f_{\mathrm{O}}} \cdot V_{\mathrm{E}}.$$

An objective focal length $f_{\mathrm{O}} = 200$ mm, a binocular tube focal length $f_{\mathrm{T}} = 125$ mm, and $12.5\times$ eyepieces yield a total magnification (rounded value) of

$$\frac{125 \text{ mm}}{200 \text{ mm}} \cdot 12.5 = 7.8.$$

With a given instrument constant and known magnification, the diameter of the field of view can be calculated for given microscope equipment. For details see para. 2.2.2. The diameter of the binocular tube in the intermediate image plane is said to be 20 mm. The eyepiece enlarges this intermediate image. A $10\times$ eyepiece gives the microscope user the impression of seeing an image of 200 mm diameter. This 200 mm is the above-mentioned instrument constant of Zeiss operation microscopes. The diameter of the surveyed field of view can be calculated from this value by dividing by the magnification. In the above-mentioned numerical example the value of the magnification is 7.8. The diameter of the field of view is then 200 mm/7.8 = 25.6 mm (rounded value). This relationship will again be discussed in connection with the magnification changer (section 2.4), where you will also find the complete general formula.

The choice of the eyepiece thus depends not only on the desired magnification, but also on the required diameter of the field of view. Standard power is $12.5\times$ because it offers the best compromise between magnification and surveyed field of view for the most frequently used types of microscope equipment.

b) Diopter setting. Some features of modern eyepieces facilitate their practical use. Eyepieces which bear a spectacle symbol are high-eyepoint eyepieces offering unrestricted viewing with or without spectacles. This is of special advantage to ametropic persons, because they get a correct visual impression of the environment when turning away from the operation microscope. Even more important is the ± 8 dpt * adjusting range of modern eyepieces. Within this statistically most frequent ametropic range microscope users can work without spectacles, provided their ametropia requires only spherical but not cylindrical correction of astigmatism. The value for the correction of a certain amount of ametropia is set on the eyepieces. A presbyopic person, for instance, with $+4.0$ dpt of the left and $+4.5$ dpt of the right eye sets $+4.0$ and $+4.5$ above the index lines of the left and right eyepieces. This diopter setting was also possible with older eyepiece types, but the diopter setting was often disadjusted when adjusting the microscope. The image was then blurred and fusion of the two partial images into one difficult. The problem is overcome by the spring-clip device of the new eypieces, which is released by pushing the protruding end of a rocker. The diopter value is then "locked in", the key snaps into position and disadjustment is no longer possible.

PD and diopter settings are equally important for the practical use of operation microscopes. Their correct adjustment should always be checked *before* working with the instrument.

c) Correct use of the eyepieces. When using an operation microscope one particular feature is often neglected, thus impairing its efficient use. To explain this let us return to the functional principle of operation microscopes.

---

* Diopter, abbreviated dpt. The refractive power of an optical system is the reciprocal value of the focal length. If the focal length is expressed in meters, the coefficient of the refractive power is the diopter.
Example: an objective with a focal length of $+200$ mm $= +0.2$ m has a refractive power of $1/+0.2$ m $= 5.0$ dpt.

According to para. 2.3.1, the eyepiece is used like a magnifier for re-enlargement of the intermediate image in the eyepiece tube. The intermediate image lies in the front focal plane of the eyepiece, and the eyepiece forms the enlarged intermediate image at infinity. The situation is commonly, some what inaccurately, expressed by the term

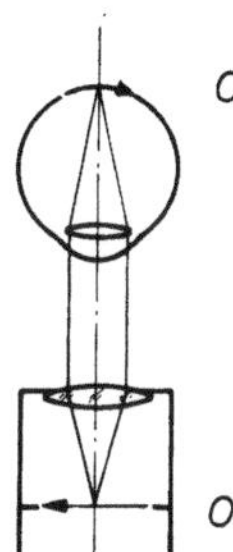

Fig. 26. The interrelationship of eyepiece and human eye (schematic). O' intermediate image plane; O'' image on the retina.

"the observation beam path is parallel behind the eyepiece". The optical system of the human eye in the parallel beam path then forms the microscopic image at a finite distance or, more accurately speaking, a sharp image is produced on the retina of a normal, non-ametropic eye (Fig. 26). The assumption that owing to the parallel beam path the distance between eye and eyepiece is of minor importance is false, as every microscopist knows, because the *illumination* beam path must be considered as well.

An operation microscope has not only one observation beam path but a combined one, i.e. observation and illumination beam paths are inseparably linked as in all compound optical systems, a fact which is often overlooked.

If an operation microscope's capabilities are to be fully utilized, the user's eyes must approach the eyepieces until the operation microscope's exit pupils lie in the planes of the user's pupils. What are the microscope's exit pupils and where are they situated? Like the observation beam path which forms an image of the object – in this case the operating field – the illumination beam path

produces an image of the light source. All operation microscopes are reflected-light microscopes, as opposed to optical microscopes for histological specimens which are used in transmitted light. In reflected light every single object point acts as a secondary light source in the illuminated operating field; it is itself a minute light source. The optical system of the operation microscope receives the light from the secondary light sources and produces an imaging illumination beam path. The operation microscope's exit pupil represents an image of the secondary light sources. The position of the exit pupil is easily found by holding a sheet of white paper into the beam path behind the eyepieces in a dimmed room. Site and lateral extension of the microscope's exit pupil are given by the narrowest point of the light bundle. The user must bring the pupil planes of his eyes to this point; only then can he fully exploit the capabilities of an operation microscope. In practice the user's eyes are quite often not near enough (for geometrical reasons the opposite case is an exception and therefore negligible) and must then accept the following two drawbacks:

I) He cannot survey the *total* field of view offered by the microscope. As if looking through a keyhole he must turn his head to change the viewing direction on the field of view. Since an operation microscope is not a monocular but a binocular stereoscopic system, many users will never get a stereoscopic impression of the object field under these conditions.

II) The second handicap is the decrease in image brightness. This becomes lower as the distance between viewing pupils and microscope exit pupils increases. This is obvious because only a fraction of the light rays coming from the microscope can reach the user's retina through his pupil. Users who are not so familiar with an operation microscope may make wrong use of the rubber eyecups, which are primarily intended to protect the user's unguarded eyes from disturbing straylight. They also help to locate the microscope's exit pupils. A user with deep-set eyes and without spectacles should always fold back the reversible eyecups so as to bring his eyes as near as possible to the eyepieces and make full use of the available light.

Spectacle wearers must always fold back the eyecups. The rubber surface prevents scratches on the spectacle lenses.

d) Frequent mistakes in the use of operation microscopes. The reasons for numerous mistakes in the use of operation microscopes and hints on their elimination have been given in the foregoing chapters. If the characteristic features of a microscope are unknown or the hints are not followed, work with an operation microscope may be tedious and unsatisfying.

As a reminder the most frequent mistakes are therefore listed again:

    I) Wrong *PD* setting of the binocular tubes.

    II) Eyepieces not completely pushed in.

    III) Wrong diopter setting of the eyepieces.

    IV) Eyepiece rubber cups not folded back where necessary.

2.3.3 Micrometer eyepieces

Micrometer disks are circular plates made of bubble- and scratch-free plate glass with a photochemically applied reticle on one side, protected by a coverglass. Depending on the magnification of the eyepiece in which the micrometer disk is used, the effective diameter varies up to max. 20 mm. The thickness of the plate is 2 mm. The micrometer disk is factory-mounted in the eyepiece so that the reticle lies exactly in the intermediate image plane. Micrometer disks are mainly applied for the following two purposes:

with scale for microscopic measurements (only in exeptional cases in operation microscopes), and more important, as a focusing aid for documentation.

a) Micrometer disks for measurement. Fig. 27 shows such an item for 12.5× eyepieces.

It has a scale from 0 to 12 graduated in intervals of 10. Before measurement this scale must be calibrated for specific microscope equipment and magnification. The simplest method with unknown microscope magnification uses graph paper as the object. The calibration procedure is explained by an

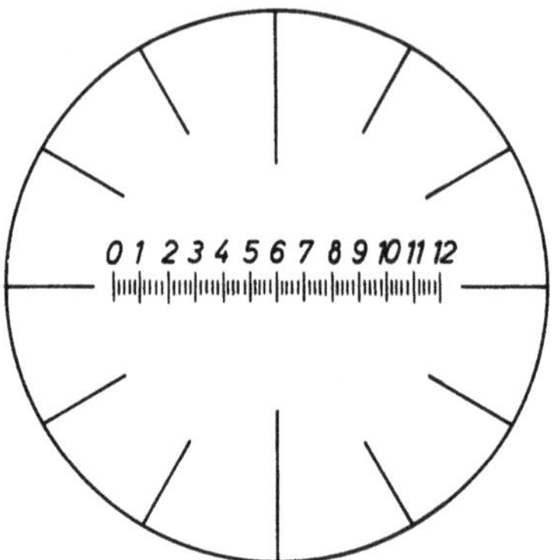

Fig. 27. Micrometer disk for 12.5 × eyepiece.

example. It is assumed that 20 mm in the object plane corresponds to 9.3 scale intervals. The calibration constant is obtained from the quotient 20 mm/9.3 scale intervals = 2.15 mm/scale interval. This value is rounded to 2.2 mm/scale interval, which is accurate enough for practical use. This determines the calibration constant for this specific type of microscope equipment. It is furthermore assumed that a measuring object in the operating field corresponds to 5.6 scale intervals of the eyepiece micrometer disk. Its actual size is the result of multiplication of this value by the calibration constant, i.e., 5.6×2.2 = 12.3 mm.

It is possible to apply a suitable, known scale directly to the measuring object in the operating field, provided a) the object is accessible, and b) the scale is sterile. This simple method is in fact used, mainly for documentation purposes. Yet the first calibration method is more universal, because it works contact-free, and can therefore also be applied in narrow body cavities.

b) Micrometer disks as focusing aids. As focusing aids these reticles are used for photographic and cine documentation. As an "instant" recording method the television technique supplies a direct, clear answer to the question of whether an interesting object field is in focus or not. Such an "instant" check is impossible in photography or cinematography through the operation microscope.

For a better understanding of why micrometer disks must be used as focusing aids for photography and cinematography through the operation micrsocope, let us go back again to Fig. 26 of para. 2.3.2 c. The picture shows the parallel observation beam path between eyepiece and observing eye. The user must look into the eyepiece with relaxed eyes as in normal distance vision. Only then are those conditions of optimum image formation fulfilled which are set by the design principle of the operation microscope. It is possible that a surgeon concentrates so intensively and exclusively on the surgical procedure that he instinctively accommodates and his eyes are no longer relaxed. As long as he alone uses the microscope and no second or even third assistant's microscope is connected, the situation is unproblematic. With an assistant's microscope, however, surgeon and assistent will not see the same object plane of the operating field in focus at the same time, unless the assistant's accommodation corresponds exactly to the surgeon's which is most unlikely. Still, during a surgical procedure surgeon and assistant can immediately contact each other and make the necessary adjustments, which is impossible during photography or cinematography. Photographic and cine equipment is so designed that the plane of the photographic emulsion corresponds *exactly* to the intermediate image plane in the eyepiece tube or, more scientifically, the plane of the photographic emulsion and the microscope's intermediate image plane are optically conjugate. By accommodation the surgeon's eyes have

adjusted themselves in the stereoscopic image in the tube to a plane other than the intermediate image plane. The image of the operating field in the intermediate image plane is then, of course, out of focus, and the image recorded on the photographic emulsion will be unsharp. This error becomes the more ob-

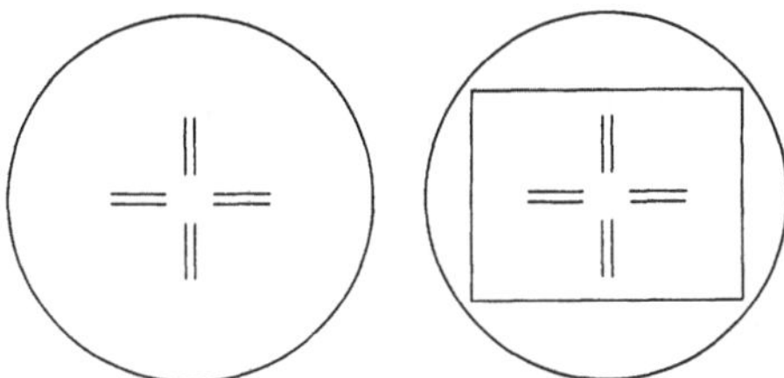

Fig. 28. Focusing aid without (left) and with format outline (right).

vious the stronger the accommodation and the higher the adjusted microscope magnification are.

These difficulties are overcome by micrometer disks as focusing aids. As mentioned before the reticle lies exactly in the intermediate image plane. For the surgeon both the selected object area and the reticle of the micrometer disk must be in focus *at the same time*. Only then will photographic or cine camera record sharp images.

Focusing plates are available with or without format outline (Fig. 28). The format outline guarantees that the photo or cine camera "sees" in fact the same section of the operating field as the surgeon has selected for recording. If not, he can adjust the microscope magnification accordingly (preferably with a magnification changer) before exposure.

Focusing aids are available for 10×, 12.5×, 16× and 20× eyepieces. The choice depends on the most suitable optical equipment for the intended application (compromise between magnification, field-of-view diameter, depth of focus and image brightness). As a rule of thumb the eyepiece (with reticle) magnification should be one step higher for documentation purposes than for normal use. Instead of a 12.5× eyepiece a 16× eyepiece is used for photography and cinematography, for the simple reason that due to the higher magnification the depth of focus is lower and the adjusting conditions of the microscope more critical.

2.4 Magnification changers

A simple, yet efficient operation microscope after Barraquer can be assembled from objectives, binocular tube and eyepieces discussed in the foregoing chapters. But many surgical procedures under an operation microscope require quick, convenient changing of the microscope magnification without modification of the microscope itself, a problem which is most elegantly solved by systems which change the magnification either in (a limited number of) steps or continuously within a certain range. Both systems are described below.

2.4.1 Galilean step magnification changer

This is the older system and the one exclusively used in the first operation microscopes. The design principle is based on the Galilean telescope which consists of a convergent objective and a divergent eyepiece. To increase the image quality, objective and eyepiece consist of cemented components instead of single lens elements. The Galilean telescope produces an upright image, and its greatest advantage is the compact design (this design principle is therefore also applied for opera glasses). In normal use the objective faces the object and the eyepiece the eye. When looking inversely through the telescope the image of a distant object will not be enlarged but reduced. Magnification changers in operation microscopes make use of this fact as will be explained below.

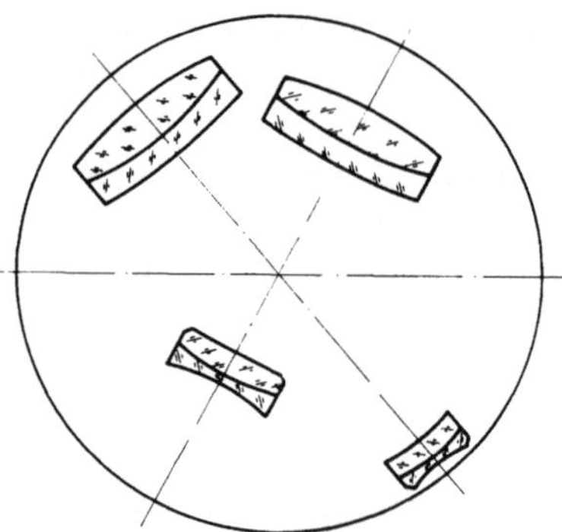

Fig. 29. Cross section (schematic) through a 5-stage magnification changer with two Galilean systems and one free path.

a) **5-stage magnification changer.** Two Galilean systems of different magnification in a drum-shaped changer that can be turned in either direction, and one additional free path (Fig. 29) allow five different magnification steps. The first telescope system has a magnification of 2.5×; in inverse use the "magnification" is 1/2.5 = 0.4. When used in both directions the second system has the magnification steps 1.6 and 0.63. Free path means that no optics are in the drum; the "magnification" equals 1. In the interest of a quick change action the free path is also provided in both directions, so that the system has actually six step positions of which two are identical. The choice of magnifications is 0.4, 0.63, 1.0, 1.6 and 2.5. Each magnification stage results from the next lower one with good approximation by multiplication by a factor of 1.6.

The 5-stage magnification changer is always integral with the microscope body. It is part of all operation microscopes of the type Opmi 1, Opmi 1 F and Opmi 1 H (details see chapter 9).

Older models of the 5-stage magnification changer carry the Figs. 6, 10, 16 (2×), 25 and 40 on the drum (Fig. 30), which refer to the total magnification of a specifically equipped operation microscope. But since microscope equipment varies considerably

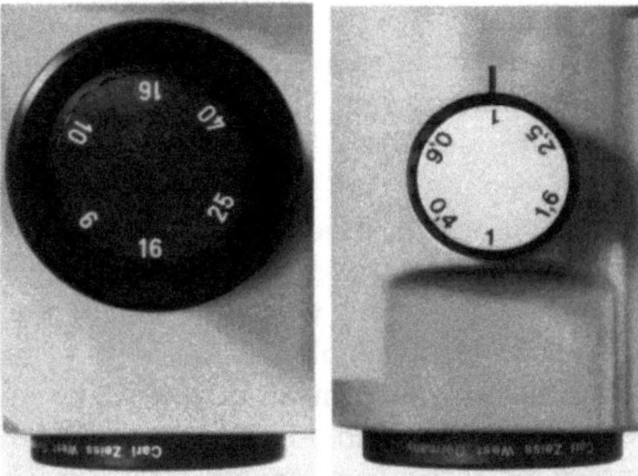

Fig. 30. Magnification selector of the Galilean magnification changer; former model (left), present, series-produced model (right).

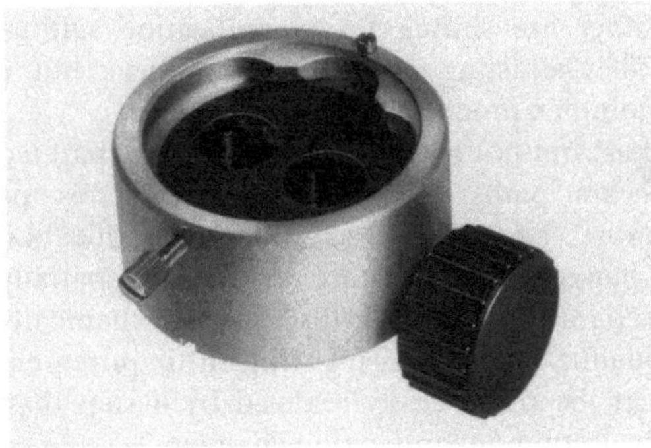

Fig. 31. 3-stage Galilean magnification changer as separate unit.

even within one and the same discipline, indication of the total magnification is misleading. New systems therefore bear only the actual magnification factor, unchanged since 1953. Table 2 lists the former values and the new magnification factors.

Table 2. Figures on 5-stage magnification changers of Zeiss operation microscopes

Old	6	10	16	25	40
New (actual magnification factor)	0.4	0.63	1.0	1.6	2.5

The magnification factor set is indicated by an index line above the drum.

b) 3-stage magnification changer. This system has only one Galilean system, one free path, and the magnification steps 0.63, 1.0 and 1.6 (Fig. 31). Other than the 5-stage changer this one is not built in but an independent module which is preferably used in the basic equipment of simple microscopes such as the operation microscope after Barraquer, the Opmi 9 diagnostic microscope and all assistant's microscopes. The 3-stage system attaches also to older instruments and supplies satisfactory results. The three steps of the changer are not specifically marked.

2.4.2 Zoom magnification changers

Step magnification changers have been proven elements of operation microscopes for more than two decades, and are still greatly appreciated because of the following major advantages:

   I) Compact design.
  II) Little technical outlay.
 III) High economy.
 IV) High optical performance.
  V) Wide magnification range from 0.4× to 2.5×.
 VI) Stepwise magnification change which is adequate for many applications.

The first series-produced operation microscope with zoom magnification changer [9c, 9e] came on the market in 1966 (Fig. 32). Apart from the magnification change being in steps or continuously variable, there are the following fundamental differences between the two systems.

A step magnification changer is no more and no less than a small telescope, and a telescope can be optimally dimensioned and manufactured with respect to image quality. The second magnification is a present due to the telescope's inverted use, and does not require thorough additional thought (this applies to the observation but only partly to the illumination beam path).

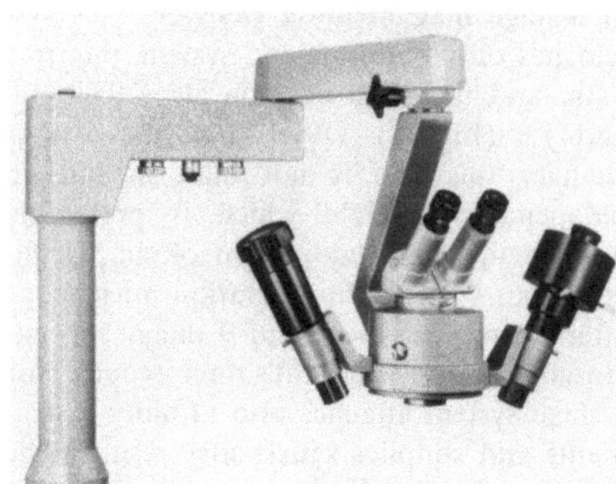

Fig. 32. The first Zeiss operation microscope with zoom system (Opmi 2).

A second telescope in the magnification changer is like the first one an enclosed system which must only meet the marginal condition that its magnification should differ from that of the first system by a factor of 1.6.

Under these conditions the free path of the magnification changer can be considered a "third system", or a system which supplies a magnification step without optics.

The 5- and the 3-stage magnification changers – the first even more than the second – are good examples of how a well thought-out combination of just a few items forms an efficient module which can be most economically utilized. It is in this sense that the term "economy" is used under III) above. While step magnification changers are not difficult to compute and design, the same does not apply to zoom magnification changers.

Zoom magnification changers must cover the entire magnification range from 0.5× to 2.5×, for instance, by *one* single optical system. Correction of image aberrations must be of a very high standard over the entire magnification range, and last but not least a zoom system must maintain the focal plane set on the microscope.

Besides extremely high demands on the zoom magnification changer itself it must

also function properly in combination with the various modules and accessories of the operation microscope. These complex problems with regard to the optics of zoom systems can only be solved by electronic computers, which delayed the appearance on the market of the first zoom operation microscope till 1966, when the first large computers were available.

All mechanical parts must, of course, be of the same high standard. A zoom system consists of three components (see Fig. 33 and para. a) of this section). Each of these components is a compound system of two cemented lens elements. The component facing the eyepiece is fixed, while the two other are shiften for magnification setting. The adjusting motion is not linear but a complex function following a curve.

Last but not least the two spatially separated beam paths of the operation microscope must be considered. The magnification changer must therefore include two spatially separated yet optically and mechanically identical systems. This stringent requirement can be more easily realized by a step than by a zoom magnification changer.

The subject of design principle and technology of zoom systems has been dealt with in some detail. If this helps to convince the user of an operation microscope that the instrument needs special care, the comprehensive explanations have served the purpose well.

Operation microscopes with 5-stage magnification changers are a familiar sight in operating theaters the world over used by virtually all disciplines of microsurgery; they have remained to this day a classic and are still a frequent choice. Why are then zoom microscopes, which require such a great technical outlay built at all? Zoom systems are not made because they are just the "rage", or to follow a general trend towards "modern" microscopes. This would be a misinterpretation of their importance. For a number of important reasons zoom microscopes are absolutely necessary for many practical applications. Operation microscopes are widely used in microsurgery also because of the ample selection of co-observation and documentation equipment. With the aid of a zoom magnification system a selected image area is fully utilized for photographic or cine recording. After a general survey of the total operating field the zoom system permits a swift change to the actually required area.

Another great advantage is that the action of a zoom magnification changer can be motorized and foot-panel controlled, which frees the surgeon's hands completely for microsurgery. This last point is the more important the more sophisticated the surgical technique.

With a zoom magnification changer the user can continuously survey the operation field, even during adjustment, a feature which cannot be realized by a step magnification changer.

Since with a motorized zoom system the operation microscope's most frequently operated functions – focusing and magnification change – are foot-panel controlled, the microscope need not be touched during surgical treatment, and may even be insterile; at least its sterility does not require the usual attention.

These facts explain the great success of zoom systems in microsurgery. Zoom microscopes have become indispensable pieces of equipment in many fields of application.

a) Zoom system 1:5. The operating principle is shown schematically in Fig. 33. Magnifications between 0.5× and 2.5× are obtainable when the movement of the central component follows a curve (Fig. 34). The left component must be shifted simultaneously. The system has a zoom factor of 5 because the maximum magnification (2.5×) is 5-times higher than the basic magnification (0.5×).

Fig. 34 shows the symmetrical zoom magnification changer with the double system for both observation beam paths. Except for the electrical connections for the zoom motor power supply, the assembly group is ready for mounting in the microscope.

Fig. 35 shows an Opmi 6 operation microscope with built-in zoom magnification

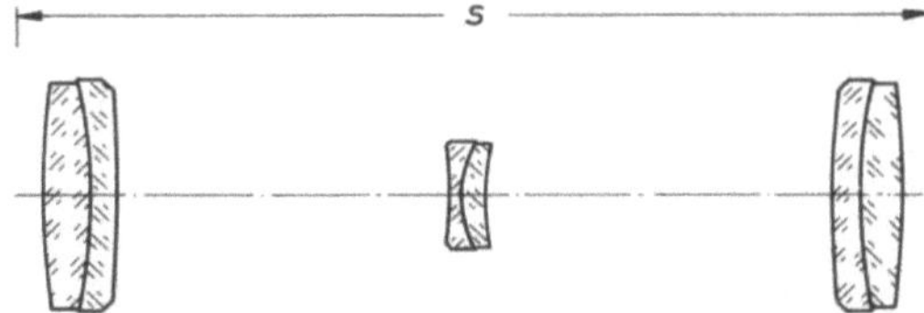

Fig. 33. Function of the zoom system (schematic). *s* shifting space.

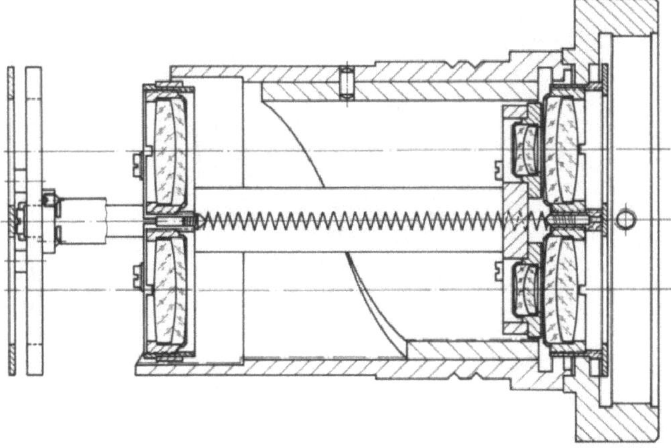

Fig. 34. The complete assembly group of the zoom system.

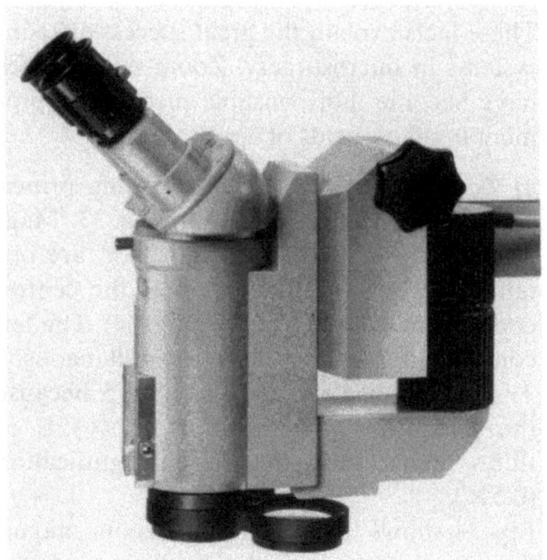

Fig. 35. Opmi 6 operation microscope with built-in zoom system and objective quick changer.

changer. The zoom factor is displayed in the window beneath the index line.

b) Zoom system 1 : 4. This new zoom system has the zoom factor 4, and the magnifications range from 0.5× to 2.0×. Compared with the older 1 : 5 zoom system it does not

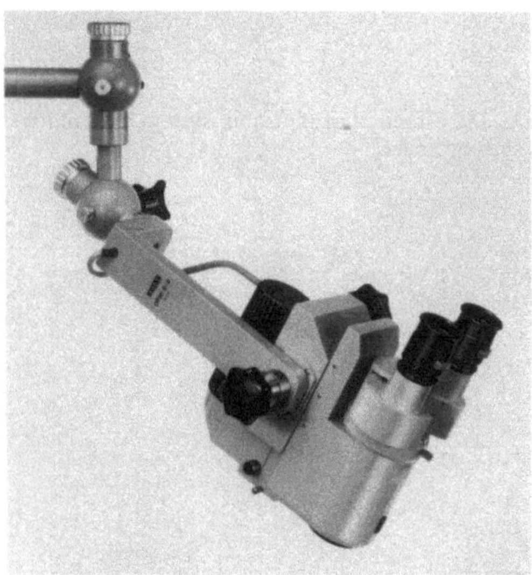

Fig. 36. Latest zoom microscope with zoom factor 4 for magnifications from 0.5 × to 2.0 × (Opmi 6 S).

mean a step backward, although it may seem like it. The new zoom system is of shorter, more compact design for which the wider magnification range is sacrificed. All other functions, the design, and the image quality in particular, correspond to those of its predecessor. This new, shorter zoom system is intended for shorter microscopes, the latest model Opmi 6 F, for instance (Fig. 36). The zoom factor is displayed in the window on the front surface of the microscope body. The motorized zoom system is provided with a manual override, a most desirable feature, for instance, in case of a power failure during an operation.

2.4.3 Parameters relating to a microscope with magnification changer

The terms magnification and field-of-view diameter have been explained in connection with the binocular tube (para. 2.2.2) and the eyepieces (section 2.3). The formulae given there apply only to microscopes without magnification changer. The formulae below are valid for all Zeiss operation microscopes with zoom or step magnification changer, and in exceptional cases even for microscopes without magnification changer (the factor of the changer must then be set 1).

a) Total magnification of a complete operation microscope. According to para. 2.3.2a the formula for the microscope magnification *without* magnification changer reads

$$\frac{f_\mathrm{T}}{f_\mathrm{O}} \cdot V_\mathrm{E},$$

where f_T is the focal length of the binocular tube, f_O the objective focal length and V_E the eyepiece magnification. Multiplication of this expression by the magnification factor of the magnification changer (for continuous and stepwise magnification change) results in the following formula for the total magnification V_M of an operation microscope:

$$V_M = \frac{f_T}{f_O} \cdot \gamma \cdot V_E \,.$$

Using the previous numerical example where $f_T = 125$ mm, $f_O = 200$ mm, $V_E = 12.5\times$, and $\gamma = 1.6$, the total magnification of an operation microscope is

$$V_M = \frac{125}{200} \cdot 1.6 \cdot 12.5 = 12.5 \,.$$

b) Field-of-view diameter of the complete operation microscope. According to para. 2.3.2 a and the preceding para a), the formula for the field-of-view diameter S_M of an operation microscope with magnification changer reads:

$$S_M = \frac{200}{V_M} \text{ mm} \,,$$

where 200 is an instrument constant and V_M the total microscope magnification. With $V_M = 12.5$ the field-of-view diameter is

$$S_M = \frac{200}{12.5} = 16.0 \text{ mm} \,.$$

c) Depth of focus of the complete operation microscope. The depth of focus is an important parameter of an operation microscope. It refers to the range within which object structures are in focus along the axis of the microscope. The limits of this range are not clearly defined, but the depth of focus can be determined for a given piece of microscope equipment by means of a formula (details see chapter 10). A surgeon is generally not interested in the microscope's depth of focus. He does not have to know it, because when he looks through the operation microscope he can see whether interesting object structures along the microscope axis are sharp enough for photographic recording, for instance. If they are not in focus he changes to a lower magnification. If he is interested in the microscope's depth of focus at a certain total magnification of the microscope, this can be obtained by a simple experiment. The depth of focus is directly determined using a small square body with a plane surface at an angle of 45°. This surface is coated with graph paper. The upper and lower limits of the range that is considered to be in focus are marked, and the distance between the two lines counted. The depth of focus is determined by dividing this value by the factor 1.4 (depths of focus of different frequently used microscopes and magnifications see chapter 10).

3 Illumination systems for operation microscopes

All operation microscopes are equipped with means to illuminate the operating field. Mostly the illumination system is rigidly connected with the microscope or is an integral part of it. External systems are offered for oblique illumination in ophthalmic microsurgery. These are in fixed position with respect to the microscope due to a common carrier. Incandescent lamps were the only light sources used in operation microscopes for almost twenty years. Today the surgeon can choose the light source which best suits his purposes from an ample selection of illumination systems. The following information is meant to assist him in his choice.

3.1 Light sources

Light sources for operation microscopes and supplementary illuminators must fulfill a number of requirements:

I) The light emission should be continuous, not intermittent.

This is not difficult to realize, because all possible incandescent and halogen light sources are continuous emitters even if run on AC voltage, which is normally used for simpler and easier power supply.

II) The light source should supply high-intensity radiation in the visible range.

The laws of physics set narrow limits to this requirement (see para. 3.1.1).

III) The light source should be economical in use.

This is possible only if it has a long life. It is not the time until it burns through which is considered the life of a lamp, but the period in which at rated voltage the intensity drops to a certain value, which varies considerably. A decrease in intensity to 70% of the initial value is for an operation microscope just about the limit that is still acceptable. As a matter of fact the technical data of lamps of one and the same type and make fluctuate considerably. The life indicated for one item does not allow conclusions to the life of this specific lamp type.

IV) The light source should illuminate the operating field uniformly.

Here the entire illumination system must be considered. Even the optically most superior illumination system correcting image aberrations to an extent usually not realized in series-produced instruments for cost reasons, will not produce satisfactory, uniform illumination when used with the wrong lamp type.

The illumination system must be fail-safe. A light source should never fail. This may happen when it is switched on, for instance, at overvoltage. The power supply should not supply overvoltage when switched on, even when previously set to it. In other words: the power supply must automatically change from overload to normal load when switched off. A lamp is also run at overvoltage if the mains voltage exceeds the rated voltage. If this is often or continually the case the voltage must be stabilized or at least the mains transformer changed by a service technician.

V) The intensity should be of adequate stability.

What is considered "adequate" depends on the application of the light source. A light source used exclusively for visual observation of the operating field is the least critical case.

It is then only necessary that its intensity does not drop *noticeably* while surgical treatment is in process. If a surgical procedure is to be documented, intensity fluctuations are allowed only for periods that can be recognized and compensated by the control unit of the documentation system. If there are no serious interferences this requirement can be fulfilled.

VI) The light source should be readily exchangeable.

If an operation microscope is equipped with only one light source this must be exchangeable without tools by the personnel in the operating theater also during a surgical procedure. Though failure of a lamp is possible its significance should not be overestimated, because two or even three external light sources are available on an operation microscope, and surgical treatment must not be interrupted.

VII) The power supply should require little technical outlay.

In addition it should be easy to operate, failsafe and simple.

VIII) The operation should be fail-safe without consideration of additional safety regulations.

This is no problem as far as incandescent and halogen sources are concerned, while high-pressure gas discharge sources are automatically excluded from use with operation microscopes. Considering the intensity they supply in the visible spectral range these last-mentioned light sources are the most desirable, but even when cold these lamps are under a pressure of 0,8 N/mm² for instance, which rises to 3 N/mm² and more when in use. They are therefore not suited for operation microscopes. Furthermore, to exchange such a lamp the user must wear face mask and gloves because of the explosion hazard.

IX) The light source should produce minimum heat.

For physical reasons additional technical outlay is necessary to guarantee this for incandescent and halogen lamps. With integral light sources unwanted high temperatures of the operation microscope during surgical procedures can only be avoided by a fan, but light sources can be set up separately in a lamp housing and connected with the microscope via fiber-optics cables (details see below).

X) The light source should be shock-proof.

The filaments of incandescent and halogen sources age due to the formation of large crystals. Vibrations which act on the lamp while in operation may then cause shearing of the filament. Operation microscopes with switched-on lamp should therefore be protected from shock or vibrations.

3.1.1 Incandescent lamps

a) The 6 V 30 W incandescent lamp has for more than two decades been the most frequent and time-tested light source of operation microscopes (Fig. 37). Rated voltage (6 V), rated power (30 W), manufacturer's serial number and the microscope manufacturer's catalog number are imprinted on the lamp. Like all others this light source does not meet the above-mentioned maximum demands, although it represents the best currently available compromise. All incandescent lamps for Zeiss operation microscopes are manufactured with prealigned snap-in sockets and need not be re-adjusted after exchange. Correctly fitted they are immediately operative.

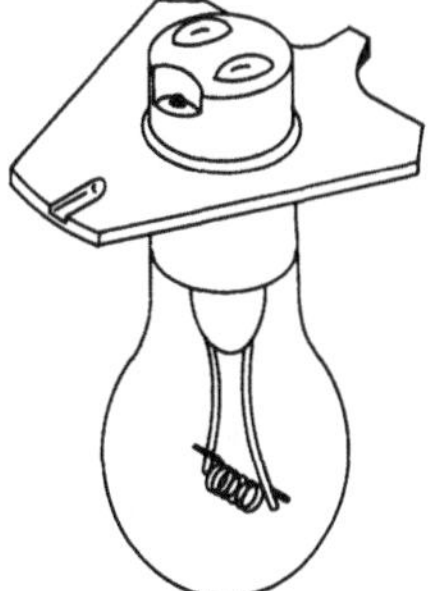

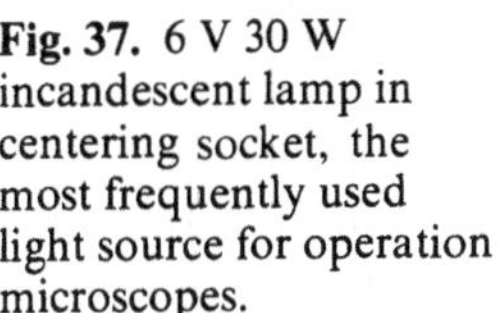

Fig. 37. 6 V 30 W incandescent lamp in centering socket, the most frequently used light source for operation microscopes.

The lamp manufacturer quotes 200 service hours as average life of the lamp at 30 W rated load. Even slight overload considerably reduces the life of the lamp. As a rule of thumb the life of a lamp is reduced to 20% if the rated voltage is exceeded by 12%. If the rated load is not exceeded too often, the 6 V 30 W lamp has a much longer life than indicated by the lamp manufacturer.

b) The 6 V 50 W incandescent lamp is a makeshift solution. In its exterior it resembles the smaller 30 W lamp, but the data are different. It is required for co-observation and documentation equipment, where higher illumination intensity of the operating field is needed than for mere visual observation, and where the intensity of the 30 W lamp is insufficient.

The heat they produce is the most serious handicap for the use of 50 W incandescent lamps in operation microscopes. It must be borne in mind that *all* incandescent lamps including the 30 W lamp, emit a maximum of only about 4% of the fed-in electrical energy as visible light. Most of the energy emission is infrared light which is invisible to the human eye. Infrared light is heat radiation. The temperature is further increased by the unavoidable heat at transfer resistances which can heat up the lamp socket to more than 200 °C. The lamp housing which is small to keep the overall dimensions of the microscope small, is also heated up to about 80 °C. Yet, even the 50 W lamp did not comply with the high demands of documentation equipment in microscopy, and was therefore frequently run at overload, often up to 50% over the rated voltage. This reduces the life of a lamp (until it breaks down completely) generally to a few hours. Only when new illumination systems were introduced were the drawbacks of these light sources overcome.

c) The 6 V 25 W incandescent lamp is used in the slit illuminator for oblique illumination in ophthalmic microsurgery. (The slit illuminator is always used together with the homogeneous illuminator. This system uses the same incandescent lamp as the integral microscope illuminator described in para. a) above.)

3.1.2 Halogen lamps

The incandescent lamps described in the preceding section have been developed for a wide voltage range. The lamp intensity is variable within wide limits by means of the voltage control and a simple potentiometer. If the lamps are run at overload to increase the intensity this shortens their lives. The intensity decreases if the lamp is run at underload and the life becomes longer.

Owing to the physical principles of their design halogen lamps are much more sensitive to over- and underload. The coil is a tungsten filament like in incandescent lamps. For a higher light efficiency the bulbs of incandescent lamps contain an inert gas, which allows higher current density and thus higher intensity. The higher current density of halogen lamps is due to the so-called tungsten-iodide cycle. Tungsten evaporates quickly at high current density, migrates to the lamp bulb where it would deposit if the wall was cool. If the temperature of all interior lamp parts is higher than 25 °C, the iodine vapor in the lamp prevents the tungsten from depositing; it diffuses back to the lamp coil as tungsten iodide. Owing to the high temperature the tungsten iodide molecules break up, tungsten deposits on the lamp coil and the iodine is released. This is why halogen lamps are more sensitive to deviations from the rated voltage: at overload or underload the tungsten iodide cycle is no longer at optimum at a certain point, the tungsten vapor deposits on the quartz bulb and reduces the light transmission for the emitted light. The lamp bulb blackens and cannot be used any more.

Halogen lamps are small, and it may be surprising that they are contained in large lamp housings. Here is the reason. Halogen lamps have a much higher light efficiency than incandescent lamps with the same power, but most of their fed-in electrical energy is also transformed into heat. The heat is eliminated either by heat conduction, that means via the lamp housing to the microscope, or by heat convection, that is again via lamp housing, and heat radiation which again puts a load on the lamp housing. Satisfactory elimination of heat for a given electrical output therefore requires certain minimum dimensions of the lamp housing and thus also of the illumination system.

There is another frequent misunderstanding with respect to the use of halogen lamps. Illuminators with halogen lamps be they built into the operation microscope or connected via flexible fiber-optics cables, are often called "coollight" illuminators, which is misleading. Halogen lamps emit a considerable portion of infrared radiation, from which the effective visible spectral range is filtered out by reflection or absorption-type heat filters. The unavoidable decrease in intensity in the visible range must be accepted.

Why are halogen lamps used in operation microscopes despite all these drawbacks, and what makes them so popular? The answer is their high color temperature. The light halogen lamps emit has a higher percentage of blue light than that of incandescent lamps. The yellow portion of the latter is greater and even tends towards red when the lamp is run at underload. The light of a halogen lamp seems to be "whiter" and thus brighter, although the objective, measured intensity difference is insignificant. The blue portion of the light generally increases the contrast of objects with different colors, and causes a more pronounced gradation of the colors.

a) The 12 V 100 W halogen lamp is either built into the operation microscope (Opmi 1 H and 6 H) or used as light source of fiber-

optics illumination systems which are discussed later. The 12 V 100 W halogen lamp (Fig. 38) – a standard light source of slide projectors – is used in operation microscopes without modification, which facilitates the spare parts supply. As shown in the diagram the lamp's longitudinal axis coincides with the axis of a parabolic mirror, so that as

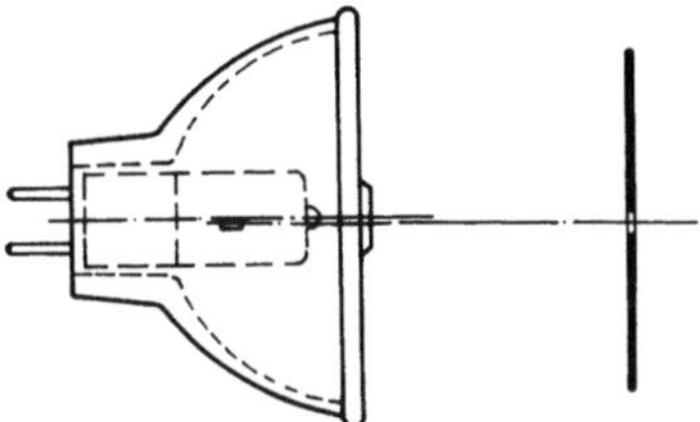

Fig. 38. 12 V 100 W halogen lamp a standard light source for slide projectors, used without modification for operation microscopes.

much of the lamp's light flux as possible is taken up and directionally radiated. The mirror also filters the incident light and separates the infrared portion from the useful visible light. For this purpose the surface of the parabolic mirror is coated with a thin metal film which gives it its reddish-violet bloom. Despite this the light rays which are radiated along the axis are not "cool" or free from infrared radiation. The 12 V 100 W halogen lamp of Opmi 1 H and 6 H is therefore used in combination with a reflection and absorption-type heat filter to suppress the infrared radiation. The manufacturer quotes 50 service hours for the halogen lamp; 10% overvoltage reduces this value to approx. 32 to 42%. At 10% undervoltage the life of the lamp is increased by a factor of 2.6 to 3.6.

b) Power supply of the 12 V 100 W halogen lamp. Fiber-optics systems as opto-mechanical connection between light source and operation microscope have the following advantages:

I) The lamp and its power supply can be mounted on the microscope stand separate

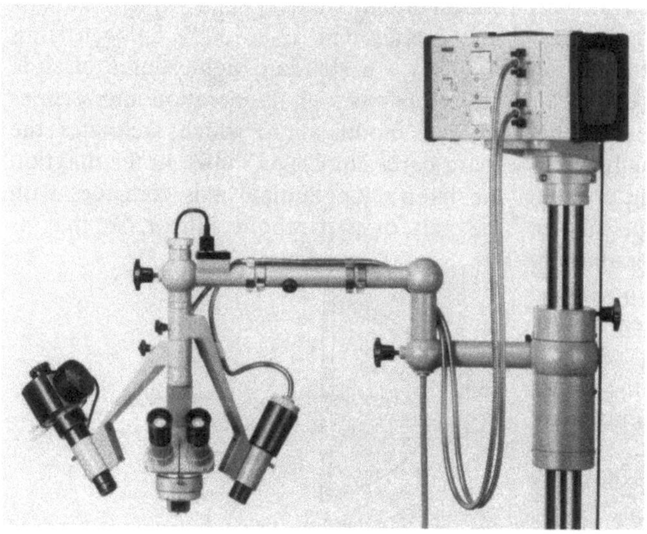

Fig. 39. Power supply for two separate fiber-optics systems, mounted on the upper end of the stand column.

from the microscope. This reduces weight and dimensions of the operation microscope, because the illumination beam path required for an integral light source is not necessary.

II) Since dimensions and weight of an external lamp housing are not as critical as those of a built-in illuminator, a double illumination system can be used. If one light source fails, switch-over to the other is a matter of seconds, but more important is the simultaneous use of both illuminators, for example for coaxial and oblique illumination (details see section 3.3).

III) The 12 V 100 W halogen lamp requires a ventilator in the microscope (or slide projector). If both illuminators are in use a high-power ventilator with high air throughput per unit of time must provide the necessary cooling. It can be included in the power supply unit.

IV) Last but not least the stringent safety regulations of some countries are complied with if the power supply unit is mounted at the upper end of the stand.

Fig. 39 shows the front view of the power supply of two external illuminators. The ventilator works if the on-off switch is on. The noise of the running ventilator is unavoidable but not disturbing. It increases slightly if both lamps are run at full load. In normal use the lamps are run at a supply voltage below rated voltage; their life is then longer than indicated by the manufacturer. At the next higher voltage stage both lamps run at rated load. The lamps are easily exchangeable without tools. The lamp socket snaps into position and no further adjustment is necessary (Fig. 40).

3.2 Light-transfer systems

The opto-mechanical coupling of illuminator and operation microscope, be it simple or complex, must meet certain requirements.

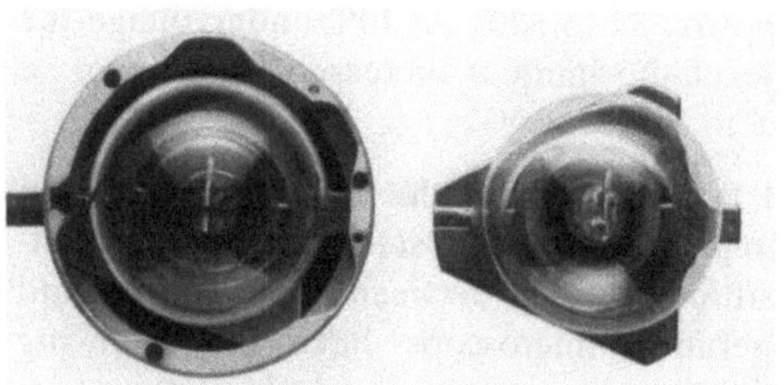

Fig. 40. No tools are required for the lamp exchange.

3.2.1 Integral illumination systems

a) Illumination beam paths of Opmi 1, 6, and 9. These three microscopes (Opmi 9 is more a piece of diagnostic equipment than an operation microscope) have the same illumination beam paths (diagram see Fig. 41). The light is relayed through the lamp condenser via a deflecting prism and a color filter to the heat filter, and via a further deflecting prism (illuminating prism) of additional convergent power through the microscope objective to the operating field. Two conditions of image formation must be fulfilled:

I) The lamp condenser produces an enlarged image of the lamp coil in the exit opening of the illuminating prism. Only when this opening is completely and uniformly illuminated, is the maximum effective intensity of the luminous field (the circular illuminated area of the operating

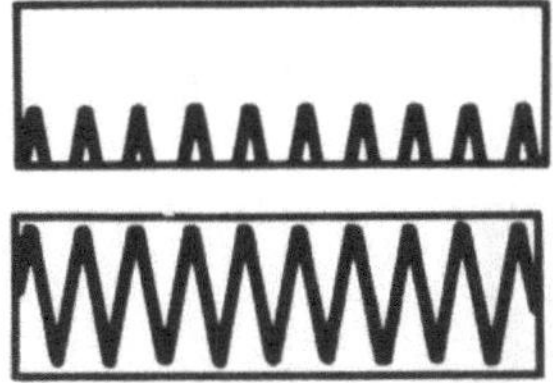

Fig. 42. In case of a defective lamp the image of the lamp coil does not completely cover the exit opening of the illuminating prism (above) and only part of the maximum available intensity is utilized. Centered image of the lamp coil (below).

field) achieved. At a lower image scale of the lamp condenser (and otherwise unchanged conditions) only part of the prism's exit opening is illuminated, and the brightness decreases. If despite optimum dimensions of the optical system only part of the illuminating prism is covered by the enlarged image of the lamp coil, this is due to a defect. The soldering metal of the pre-aligned lamp socket melts if it is not heat-resistant enough, and the spring pressure which acts on the socket and keeps the lamp in a defined position, shifts the lamp coil from its center position; it is decentered (Fig. 42).

A higher image scale of the coil image would not bring about higher light intensity of the operating field because the intensity does not increase if the coil image is larger than the exit prism, but reflections in the observation beam path may considerably impair the image contrast. To avoid this, the lamp coil image should not completely cover the illuminating prism. Even in the most unfavorable case the coil image reaches only as far as a prism edge owing to the unavoidable tolerance fluctuations of the lamp coil position. In older operation microscopes the prism edge is protected by a lacquer coating

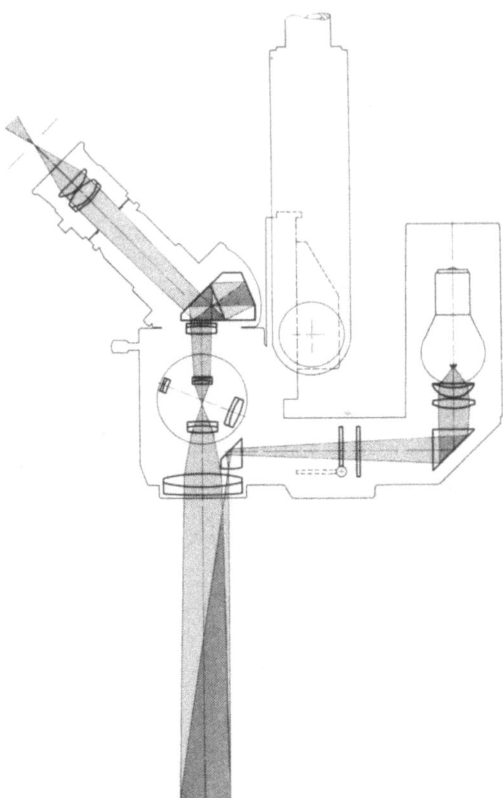

Fig. 41. The classical illumination beam path of the operation microscopes Opmi 1 and Opmi 6 and of the diagnosis microscope Opmi 9.

to suppress reflections (Fig. 43). If the lamp coil image is decentered, a loss in intensity is likely to occur.

II) According to the second requirement of image formation the convergent illuminating prism must form an image of the lamp condenser aperture on the operating field. It defines the luminous field of the operating

Fig. 43. To avoid reflections the edges of the illuminating prism of older operation microscope models are provided with a lacquer coating.

field. This requirement is less problematic than the first, because the parameters are unambiguously defined and not subject to variations as, for instance, the position of the lamp coil.

If the above-mentioned requirements are fulfilled, the illumination beam path is in accordance with Köhler's rules, which means the luminous field is uniformly illuminated with reasonable intensity and sharply defined. Even if on a white sheet of paper the outlines of the lamp coil image are visible, this is negligible for operation microscopes because this image is invisible in the operating field. It is due to the way the filament is coiled but not to defects of the optical system in the illumination beam path.

Besides the above-mentioned advantages the Köhler illumination principle has another important one: the illumination beam path comes up to the microscope objective and must never be changed, not even after objective exchange. With every new objective the illumination system "automatically" provides uniform, high-intensity, sharply defined illumination of the luminous field. The instrument manufacturer generally provides for a diameter of the luminous field which is larger than that of the field of view, because only then is the microscopic image illumi-

nated to the very edges. At very low magnifications of the operation microscope, however, the diameter of the field of view may be larger than that of the luminous field as, for instance, shown in Fig. 44. The problem can be solved by a supplementary illuminator. For some applications in neurosurgery or otorhinolaryngology a smaller

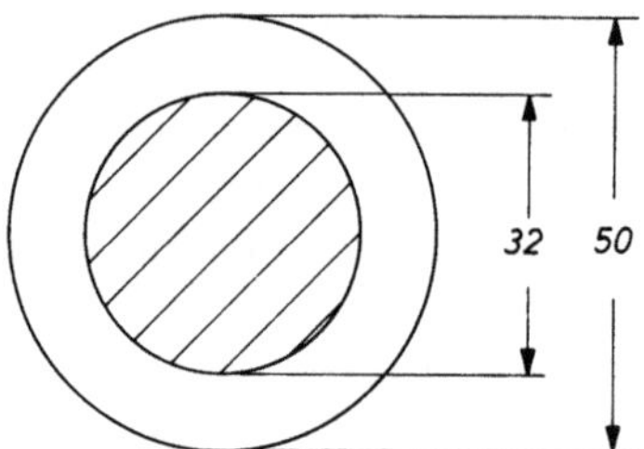

Fig. 44. At extremely low magnifications of the operation microscope the field-of-view diameter may be larger than the diameter of the luminous field. $\beta = 4 \times$, $f = 200$, $f_T = 160$, eyepiece 12.5 ×, changer position 6 × (0.4).

luminous field is preferred to avoid disturbing light and to enhance the contrast. The illumination system described below includes an adjustable iris diaphragm in the illumination path for this purpose.

Table 3 lists the luminous field and field-of-view diameters of some frequently used microscope types.

Table 3. Luminous field and field-of-view diameters of frequently used microscope types with binocular tube $f = 125$ mm and 12.5 × eyepieces.

	175	200	400
Objective focal length [mm]	175	200	400
Luminous field diameter [mm]	28	32	64
Field-of-view diameter [mm] in position 16 of magnification changer	18	20	25

b) Illumination beam paths of Opmi 1 H and 6 H. The letter "H" stands for the built-in halogen lamp, the figure "1" or "6" for a 5-stage or zoom magnification changer. The illumination beam path of both microscope types are identical. The schematic side view shows that the design principle is the same as that of the microscopes Opmi 1, 6, and 9 described in the preceding paragraph (Fig. 45). Only the differences are dealt with in this paragraph. The high output of the lamp of 100 W calls for ventilation of the

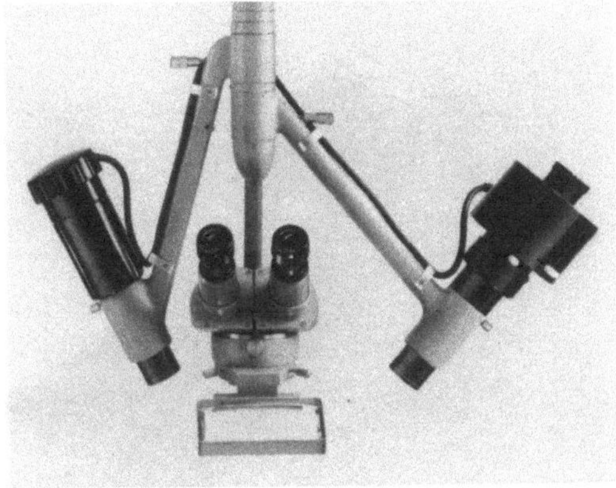

Fig. 45. Homogeneous illuminator (left) and slit illuminator (right) on operation microscope Opmi 3 equipped with additional operating field magnifier.

lamp housing. The noise of the built-in ventilator is audible but not disturbing; it becomes louder as the lamp voltage rises. The exhaust air is angulated upwards away from the operating field to avoid contamination of this area.

Easily exchangeable color filters can be brought into the beam path in a filter slider.

An iris diaphragm in the lamp condenser plane allows continuous change of the luminous field diameter from max. 40 mm with $f = 200$ mm objective to half this value.

The microscopes 1 H and 6 H have the following major advantages:

I) The high-intensity white light of the halogen lamp is superior to incandescent lamp illumination for all kinds of microsurgery because of the high contrast it produces. However, but they should not be used in ophthalmology.

II) A red-free (green) filter for contrast enhancement will always cause a light loss. Owing to the brightness reserve this is more acceptable with a halogen than with an incandescent lamp.

III) At high magnifications which are the rule in vascular surgery incandescent lamps are soon at the limit of their capacity; not so the light sources of Opmi 1 H and 6 H.

IV) The microscopes Opmi 1 H and 6 H are most favorable for co-observation and documentation. Documentation equipment (described in chapter 8) will always bring about light losses, but these are more than compensated by the 100 W halogen lamp. It also permits the use of a small aperture stop in the photo, cine or TV adapter, which results in a greater depth of focus.

c) **Special illuminators for ophthalmic microsurgery.** Surgical procedures such as corneal transplants or cataract extractions require high-efficiency illumination systems of the operation microscope. Direct, coaxial illumination which will be discussed later is not suitable for this kind of work, because of disturbing reflections which not only bloom the entire microscopic image, but may also lead to temporary blind spots in the surgeon's visual field. In clear media details can be made visible only by means of light scattering. Different types of external inclined illumination systems have therefore been developed for ophthalmic microsurgery.

Homogeneous and slit illuminator (Fig. 45) are always used in combination. The homogeneous (to the left in the figure) and the slit illuminators form angles of 27° and 35° with the vertical axis of the operation microscope; both illuminators are rotatable around a common vertical axis. The above angles are valid for an objective focal length of 175 mm. In this position the homogeneous illuminator produces at the appropriate distance a circular luminous field of 45 mm diameter. Owing to the inclined axis direction of the lamp the luminous field is deformed into an

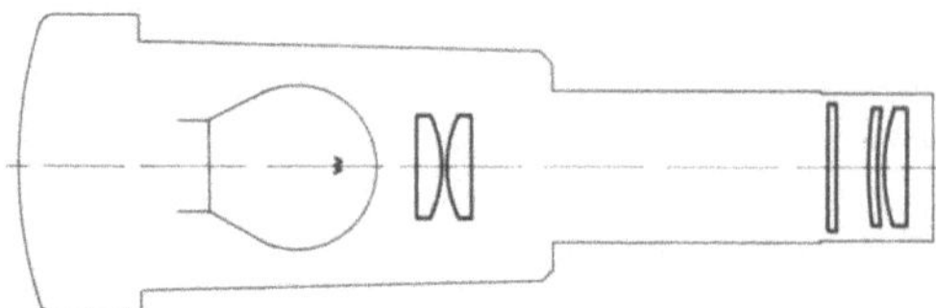

Fig. 46. Design and beam path of the homogeneous illuminator.

ellipse in the case of a flat object plane. This fact is negligible if the object has a spherical front surface like the eye. The term "homogeneous illuminator" indicates that, contrary to the slit illuminator, it illuminates an extensive field homogeneously, and can be applied for illumination of the entire operating field. Its technical concept corresponds to the above-mentioned principles of illumination beam paths in operation microscopes (Fig. 46).

The slit illuminator is equally important and indispensable for ophthalmic microsurgery. It produces in the operating field a slit image of variable width (0 to 20 mm, that is the full circular aperture) and three different heights. The slit illuminator is designed for Köhler illumination (Fig. 47). The slit assembly is arranged next to the lamp condenser plane to guarantee a sharply defined image of the slit outlines in the operating field. Homogeneous and slit illuminator are rotatable around the microscope's vertical axis. This motion alone is insufficient for

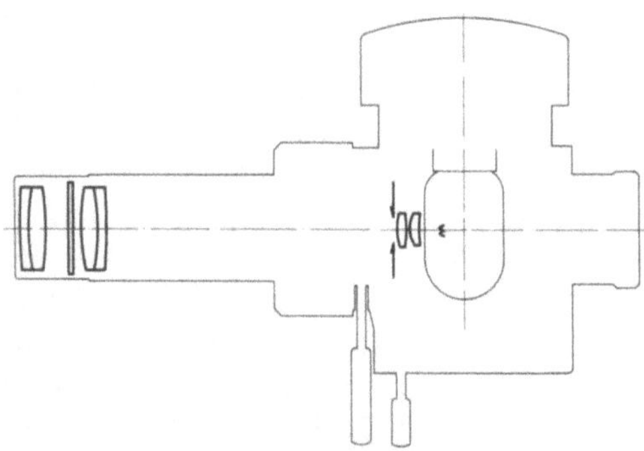

Fig. 47. Design and beam path of the slit illuminator.

optimum utilization of the slit illuminator. The slit must also be adjustable ± 10 mm to either side from center position, which is achieved by a supplement (Fig. 48) that can be subsequently slipped onto the lower sleeve of the slit illuminator and secured. The slit image is adjusted by means of a

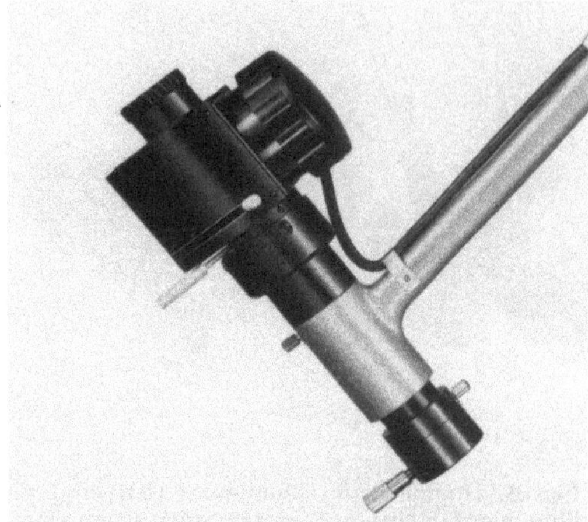

Fig. 48. Supplement for slit illuminator to adjust the slit image ± 10 mm to either side from the center position.

knurled screw which can be covered by a sterilizable metal cap. The luminous fields of homogeneous and slit illuminator must be centered, that means aligned with the focal length of the microscope objective. This adjustment is made with the corresponding lamp carrier and is not described in this connection.

The ± 30° slit illuminator (Fig. 49) is needed above all for vitreous surgery. Illumination and observation are realized via a three-mirror contact lens, so that there is only a reduced solid angle for adjustment of the slit illumination. The slit illuminator described in the preceding paragraph cannot be used because of the large and invariable angle it forms with the microscope axis. The new, motorized, ± 30° slit lamp is adjustably mounted on an arc below the microscope.

The illuminator is permanently aligned to the microscope's $f = 175$ mm objective working distance, and can be rotated continuously from 30° left to 30° right of the microscope's vertical optical axis. This range seems rather wide, but the illuminator is also used for work without contact lens, that is

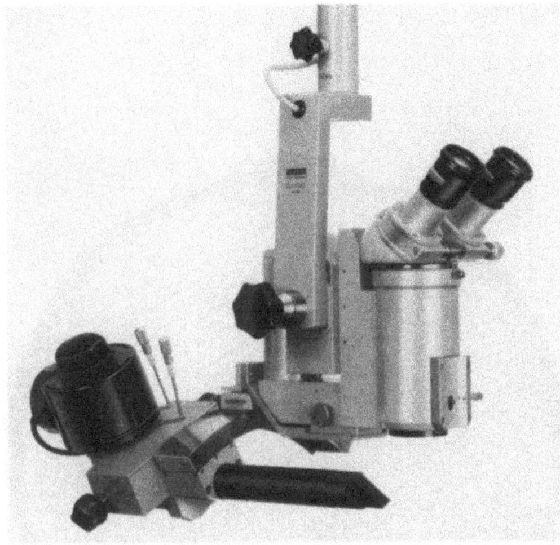

Fig. 49. The ± 30° operation slit illuminator mounted on an arc below the zoom microscope Opmi 6.

for surgery of the anterior media of the eye or for diagnostic purposes which require efficient slit lamp illumination of recumbent patients. The design is shown in Fig. 50. The beam path is in accordance with the rules of Köhler illumination, but the optical components are different. Homogeneous, slit and ± 30° slit illuminators have different optical systems. Some technical data of the ± 30° slit illuminator which are important for the surgeon: motorized movement (approx. 5°/s), remote-controlled by foot panel, with manual override as a fail-safe; 6 V 25 W incandescent lamp, swing-in green filter for contrast enhancement; continuously variable slit width from 0 to the full 9 mm dia. circular aperture; six slit heights of 9, 7, 5, 3.5, 2.5, and 0.3 mm; slit rotation by rotation of the lamp housing; extended levers for slit width and slit height adjustment can be provided with sterilizable, plug-on metal caps; mounting by means of dovetails, exchangeable in seconds without re-adjustment.

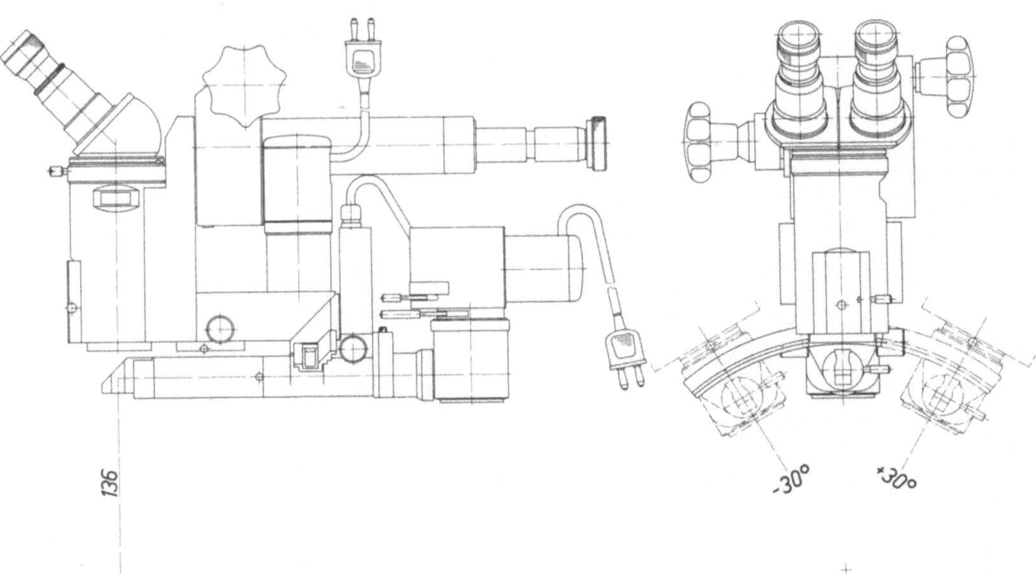

Fig. 50. Mount and adjusting range of the ± 30° operation slit illuminator

3.2.2 Fiber-optics systems

Modern fiber-optics systems for all kinds of illumination are also applied for the opto-mechanical coupling of external light sources and an operation microscope. As a reminder of the advantages of fiber-optics systems the most important features are listed again:

I) The lamp housing does not transfer heat to the microscope body.

II) The lamp housing can be installed at a distance from the microscope, i.e. at the upper end of the stand; it can be so dimensioned as to accept two light sources. If one lamp fails switch-over to the other is a matter of seconds; two separate light sources can also be used at a time.

III) Depending on design and application, fiber-optics systems can be subsequently fitted to available microscopes. The design of an operation microscope specifically developed for fiber-optics illumination will be more compact.

IV) Fiber-optics systems permit coaxial (para. 3.3.1) and oblique illumination (para. 3.3.2).

Unfortunately these systems have disadvantages, too:

I) They are technically more sophisticated and therefore more expensive than built-in illumination systems.

II) Fibers may break if a cable is bent sharply. This will reduce the efficiency of light transmission and increase light losses.

III) Even if no fibers are broken, light losses are unavoidable at the point where the light is fed in: it is typical for the intensity to be reduced to half its value.

IV) Color filters are difficult to bring into the beam path.

V) The light loss due to absorption is the higher the longer the fiber-optics cable.

The fiber-optics systems for operation microscopes were chosen from the wide choice that is on the market with the special intention of minimizing the above-mentioned disadvantages. Fig. 51 shows a fiber-optics

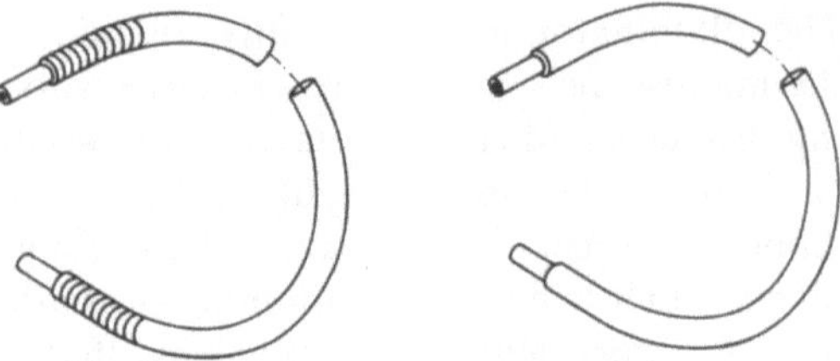

Fig. 51. Fiber-optics cable for operation microscopes.

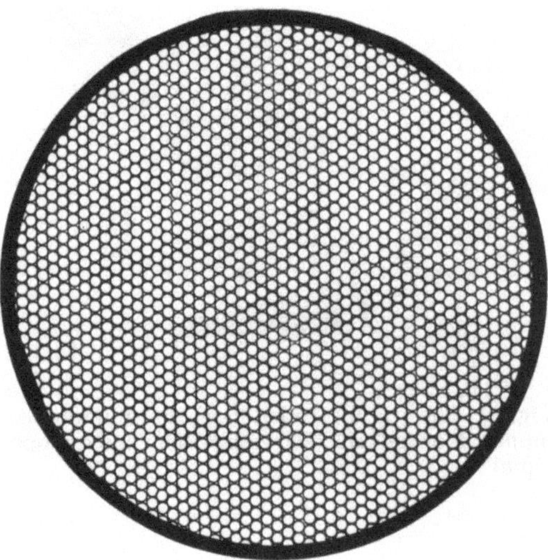

Fig. 52. Entrance opening of fiber-optics cable.

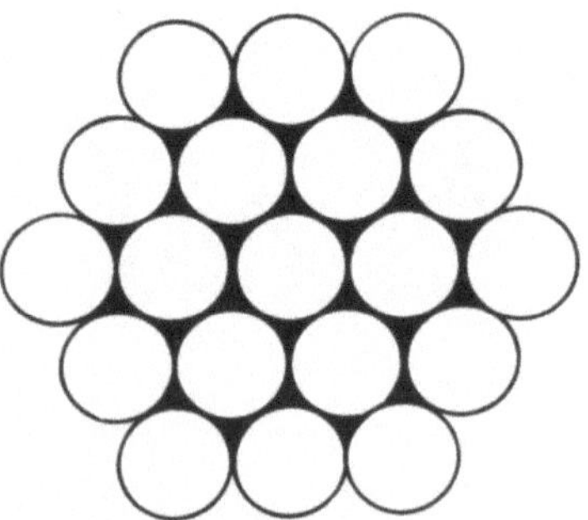

Fig. 53. The black areas show the loss due to empty spaces between the fibers at the entrance opening of the fiber-optics cable.

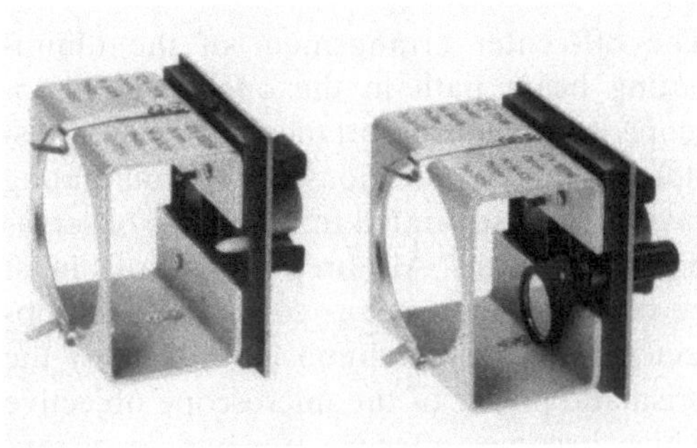

Fig. 54. A color filter in the illumination beam path with fiber-optics system.

cable in a metal tube to protect the fibers, Fig. 52 a cable end. The cable's effective diameter is 8 mm, and the diameters of the individual fibers are usually 0.020 mm. The single fibers have circular cross sections. If they are combined in cables there are empty spaces between the fibers, where no light is transmitted; they cause the above-mentioned 50% light loss. Fig. 53 explains this schematically. As said before, it is difficult to bring color filters into the beam path of illumination. The best place for a color filter would be in the lamp housing in front of the entrance opening of the fiber-optics system (Fig. 54). But at this place the filter would be exposed to strong heat, and absorption-type color filters which are normally used in operation microscopes are very heat-sensitive and would break. Only heat-resistant color filters can be used. To check a fiber-optics cable for broken fibers which cause light losses the operation microscope itself is used: the cable is shifted axially from the optimum, factory-adjusted position until the individual fibers are visible in the image plane (Fig. 55). It will be necessary to exchange the cable if too many fibers are broken.

3.3 Types of illumination

The hints given in this section are meant to help the surgeon find the illumination system which best suits his purposes. Some previous statements must be repeated for the sake of completeness.

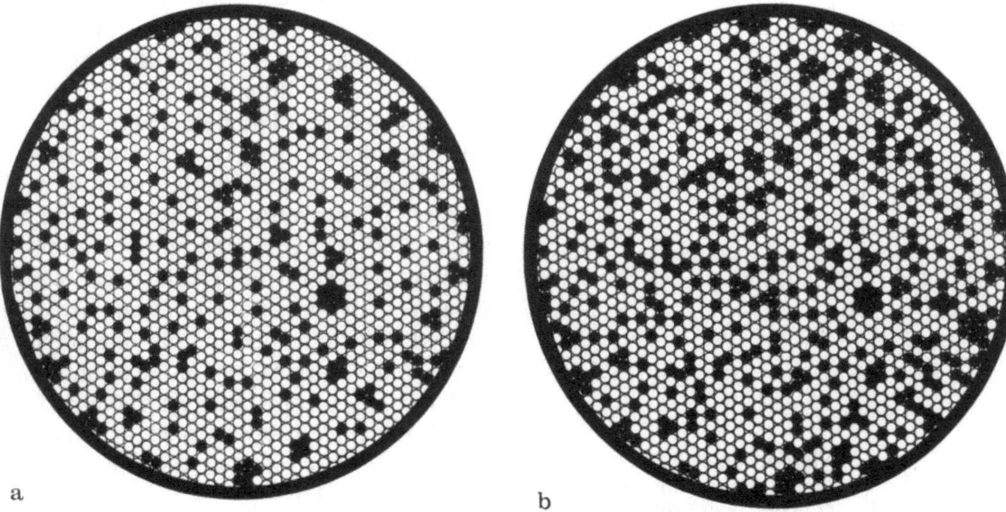

a
b

Fig. 55. Checking a fiber-optics cable for broken single fibers. 15% of the fibers are broken in a, 25% in b. In the latter case the cable must be replaced.

3.3.1 Coaxial illumination

a) Principle. In the strictest sense of the word the illumination beam path for coaxial illumination of the operating field would have to be guided through the microscope along the microscope axis. But this is neither possible nor desirable. According to Figs. 56 and 57 of para. 2.1.5 the diameter of each of the two observation beam paths is 16 mm, and the distance between the two center points 22 mm. It follows for the (assumed) illumination system that its width would be only 6 mm, a value which would have to be even further reduced to avoid reflections (see para. 3.2.1). Another stipulation is that the illuminating prism should be as large as possible and fully covered by the image of the lamp coil to guarantee maximum light intensity in the operating field. The illuminating prism is therefore arranged off-center *next to* the two observation beam paths. Such an arrangement is strictly speaking "quasi-coaxial", but the term "coaxial illumination" has meanwhile become so popular that it is retained here.

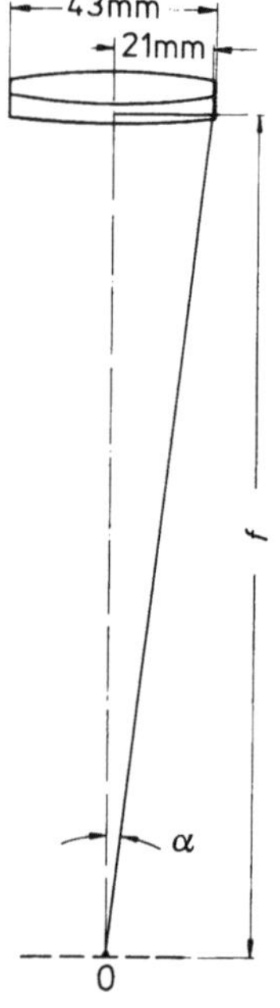

Fig. 56. Angle α between marginal illuminating ray and microscope axis, referred to the center of the field of view in the object plane *O*.

The off-center arrangement of the illuminating beam path in the operation microscope is of great importance for the suppression of direct reflections. The illuminating rays are well separated from the two observation beam paths. All three beam paths must be centered, that means coincide in the object plane. This condition is fulfilled by the prismatic power of the microscope objective which becomes effective if a bundle of rays passes off center.

b) Angle separating illumination and observation. Fig. 56 explains how the illumination beam path and the two observation beam paths are separated in their upper parts, and how completely they coincide in the object plane (lateral view).

The illustration also shows that the illumination beam path is off center but the axis of the illuminating bundle not too far away from the microscope axis, because the diameter of the microscope objective is only 43 mm. The illuminating prism lies within the objective's diameter, and its outer edge can therefore only be at a distance of about 21 mm from the objective center. For the shortest objective focal length of 175 mm, the ratio of 21/175 yields an angle of 6.9° subtended by the marginal ray of the illumination and the microscope axis. This is so small an angle that it also justifies the use of the term "coaxial illumination".

An extremely small angle between illumination and microscope axis is a pre-condition for surgery in narrow, deep operating fields (surgery of intravertebral disks, intercranial surgery, larynx and tympanum operations or vitreous surgery). Here greater focal lengths then the above-mentioned 175 mm are often needed, which further reduce the angle α between the marginal ray of the illumination and the microscope axis. At 200 mm focal length the angle α is only 6.0°, at 300 mm it decreases to 4.0°, and at 400 mm objective focal length to 3.0°.

These examples show that a shorter distance between the microscope's illumination beam

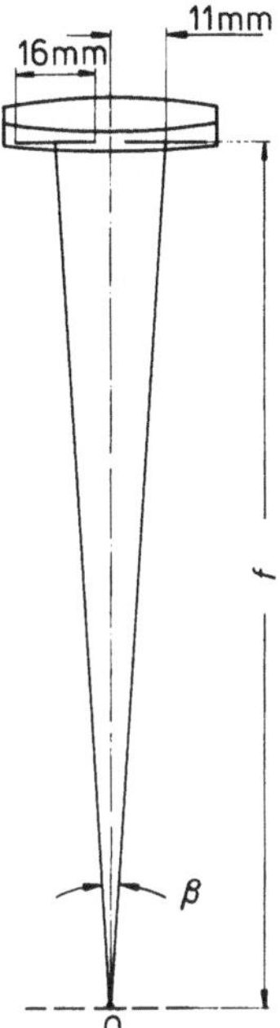

Fig. 57. Angle β between the centers of both observation beam paths of the objective, referred to the center of the field of view O.

path and the microscope axis is not necessary. The distance between the axes of the two observation beam paths is known to be 22 mm, which almost equals the distance between the marginal ray of coaxial illumination and the microscope axis. Consequently, the angles β (Fig. 57) between the centers of the circular apertures of the two

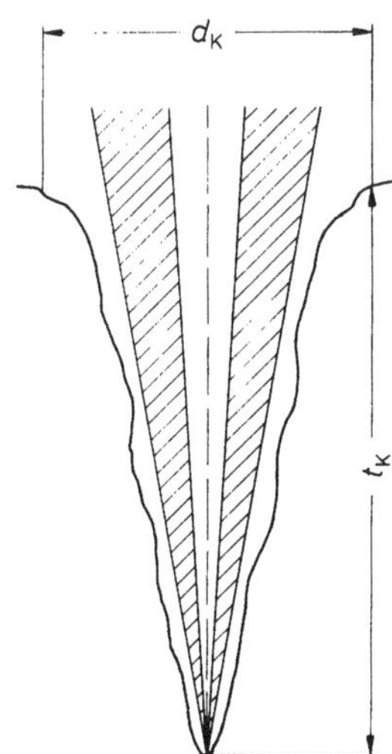

Fig. 58. Beam paths in narrow, deep cavities.

observation beam paths correspond to those of the illumination for the objective focal lengths mentioned above.

c) Narrow body cavities. Because of the fundamental importance of these considerations for surgery in narrow body cavities, some numerical examples are given. Fig. 58 is similar to Fig. 57, but the area between the marginal rays of the two observation light bundles leading to the center of the field of view is hatched. How large must the minimum diameter of a body cavity d_K be to see at the depth t_K of the body cavity the observation light bundle without cutoff with an objective focal length f? Table 4 gives the answer for the most frequently used objective focal lengths 175, 200, 300, and 400 mm. Three different values of t_K (20, 50, and 80 mm) were used for the calculation of the corresponding minimum diameters d_K of the body cavity.

Table 4. Required minimum diameter d_K of a body cavity of the depth t_K for different objective focal lengths f, without cut-off of the two observation beam paths (all values in mm, d_K values rounded)

Focal length f [mm]	t_K [mm]		
	20	50	80
175	3.9	9.7	15.5
200	3.4	8.5	13.6
300	2.3	5.7	9.1
400	1.7	4.3	6.8

According to the above table the minimum diameter d_K of the $t_K = 20$ mm deep body cavity should be 2.3 mm for an objective focal length of 300 mm. For the same objective focal length this value increases to 5.7 mm for $t_K = 50$ mm. If $t_K = 80$ mm d_K must be at least 9.1 mm, because otherwise one or even both observation light bundles would be cut off (at least partly). The actual diameters d_K must be larger than indicated in the table, because of microinstruments which would obscure the beam paths partly or completely, and because otherwise the axial and lateral adjustment of the operation microscope would be tedious and time-consuming.

d) Object-side limitation of observation beam paths. What happens if the minimum diameter d_K required for a narrow, deep body cavity according to Table 4, cannot be adhered to? Even disregarding the problem of illumination, it is unlikely that only one single observation light bundle can pass through a narrow body cavity. The depth perception or stereoscopic impression of the operating field is lost, and the operation microscope can only be used for diagnosis but not for the control of microinstruments. If both observation beam paths are partly but uniformly cut off from the outside, stereoscopic observation of the operating field at the bottom of the cavity is still possible, but the stereoscopic effect is not as pronounced as if both observation beam paths can be used without limitation. For this last case the instrument manufacturer introduced some years ago a prism system between magnification changer and objective. Its sole purpose is to reduce the stereo basis that is the distance between the two observation beam paths. For the system described here the distance between the axes of the two beam paths is 16 mm, whereas the normal value is 22 mm. This supplement did not find general approval because it reduces the image brightness.

e) Operation microscopes with coaxial illumination. Table 5 lists the operation microscopes available with coaxial illumination. Coaxial illumination systems come with incandescent, halogen, and fiber-optics sources. All illumination systems are for microscopes with 5-stage or zoom magnification changers, except for the diagnostic microscope which cannot be equipped with the 12 V 100 W halogen lamp, as it is not intended for documentation.

3.3.2 Oblique illumination on the microscope

Extreme oblique illumination, that is illumination subtending a large angle between microscope and illumination axes, is required in ophthalmic surgery for surgery of the anterior segments. Oblique illumination equipment connected with the microscope is

Table 5. Operation microscopes with coaxial illumination

Type of illumination	Microscope model		
Integral 6 V 30 W incandescent lamp	Opmi 1 5-stage magnification changer	Opmi 6 zoom microscope	Opmi 9 diagnostic microscope (3-stage magnification changer)
Integral 12 V 100 W halogen lamp with ventilator	Opmi 1 H [a] 5-stage magnification changer	Opmi 6 H [a] zoom microscope	–
Fiber-optics system with 12 V 100 W halogen lamp for supply	Opmi 1 F [b] 5-stage magnification changer	Opmi 6 F [b] zoom microscope	Opmi 9 F [b] diagnostic microscope (3-stage magnification changer)

[a] *H* stands for the built-in 12 V 100 W halogen lamp
[b] *F* stands for the integral *f*iber-optics system with 12 V 100 W halogen lamp supply.

therefore a makeshift solution, a kind of auxiliary illumination if coaxial illumination is insufficient or – for special microscope types – if there is no other type of illumination.

a) Fiber optics illumination. Fiber optics systems for oblique illumination are the latest types of illuminators directly mounted on the operation microscope. One model (Fig. 59) uses the second (of two possible) fiber optics cables as a supplement to the coaxial illumination system for better illumination of large operating fields. A carrier for two systems which can be mounted around the objective (Fig. 60) accepts either both illuminators or the conventional one only, and is used whenever a microscope has no built-in illumination system (Opmi 3, 4, 5 or 7) or if a built-in coaxial illumination system is insufficient. This may be the case in older versions of the operation microscope types 1 and 6 with 6 V 30 W lamp, for which the use of a 6 V 50 W lamp is not

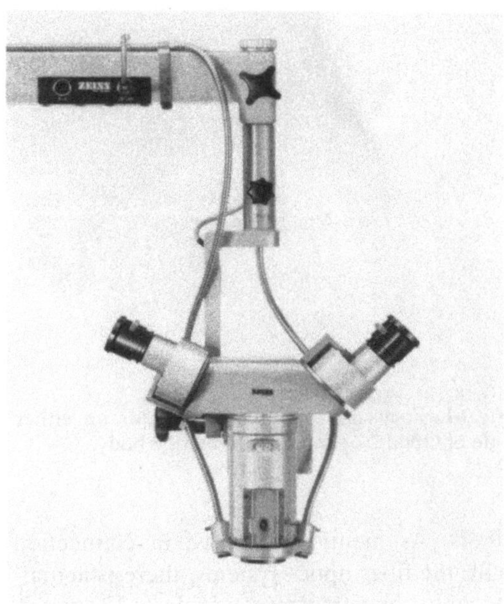

Fig. 60. Oblique tandem fiber-optics illumination system.

recommended. For a comparison of the intensities obtainable with the illumination systems described here see section 3.5.

b) Focusable illuminator. Fig. 61 shows the older version of an oblique illumination system as used in the first zoom microscope Opmi 2 [9 c], whose built-in coaxial illumination system was insufficient for co-observation. This illuminator allows optical axial focusing, i.e. after adjustment of the viewing direction with a rotatable and lockable joint the luminous field can be centered and focused on the operation microscope with microscope objectives of different focal lengths. This is impossible with inclined fiber optics illumination systems. Adjustment of the viewing direction for centering is not absolutely necessary, because the diameter of the field of view is always considerably smaller. Optical "focusing" is useless but the lower end of the fiber optics system can be shifted axially, which is useless, too, unless done to look for defective single

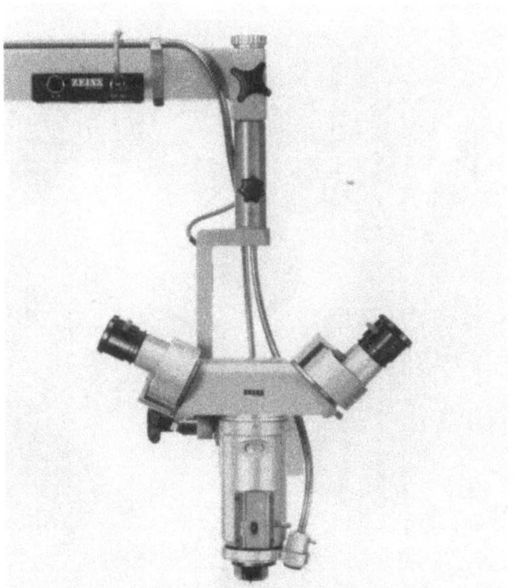

Fig. 59. Unilateral, oblique illumination on the microscope via fiber-optics cable combined with coaxial fiber-optics illumination.

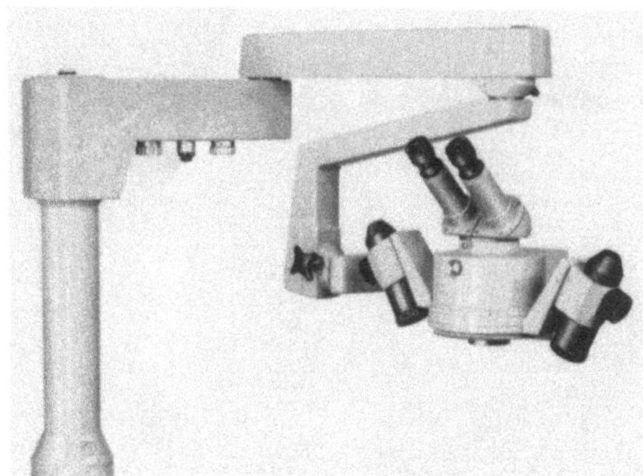

Fig. 61. Focusable oblique illuminator on either side of Opmi 2 operation microscope body.

fibers. As mentioned above in connection with the fiber optics systems, there is actually only one recommendable adjustment, where the large luminous field is homogeneous, comparatively well defined and illuminated with maximum intensity of the operating field.

This explains why the historically "old" focusable illuminator is used also on modern microscopes, unless the most efficient illumination system of the type H (with built-in 12 V 100 W halogen source) is concerned.

c) Electronic flash unit. The growing importance of co-observation and documentation a decade ago brought about the problem of how to increase the illumination intensity of the operating field. Overloading the 6 V 30 W or even the 6 V 50 W incandescent lamp was a solution only for observation. Photography required (and still does with the above-mentioned lamp types) long exposure times, which, depending on the magnification and kind of operating field could amount to some tenths of a second. The depth of focus for laryngology, for instance, requires the narrowest possible aperture in the photographic beam path. This explains the disappointing results of photographic records and the reluctant acceptance of this method by some disciplines. On the other hand it explains the early use of electronic flash units on operation microscopes.

An electronic flash automatically eliminates blurs caused by the patient, because the normal flash duration is only 2/1000 to 3/1000 s. But this almost ideal property of the flash is accompanied by two major disadvantages: in some cases not even the flash intensity supplies satisfactory illumination of the operating field, and mounting of the electronic flash below the microscope body occupies much of the working space available for surgeon and assistant. The output of electronic flashes can be increased to more than 80 Ws (of older types) and 160 Ws (of modern instruments), but this requires greater dimensions of flash unit (hardly tolerable) and power supply (possible). Despite these limitations electronic flash units are widely used, because they offer optimum photographic documentation

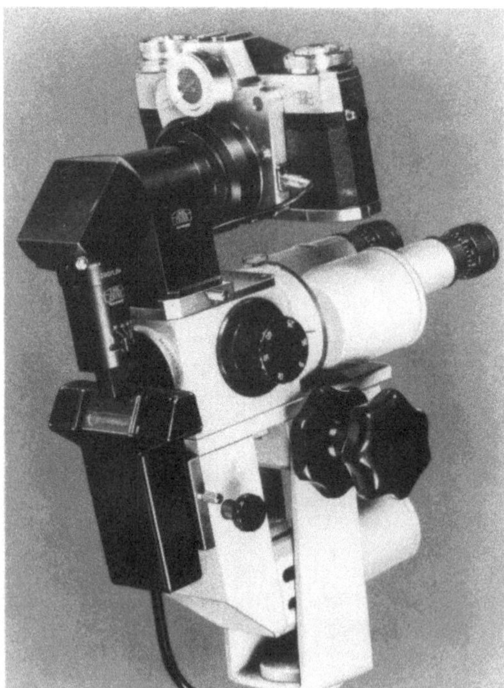

Fig. 62. Electronic flash unit on the microscope with integral coaxial illumination system.

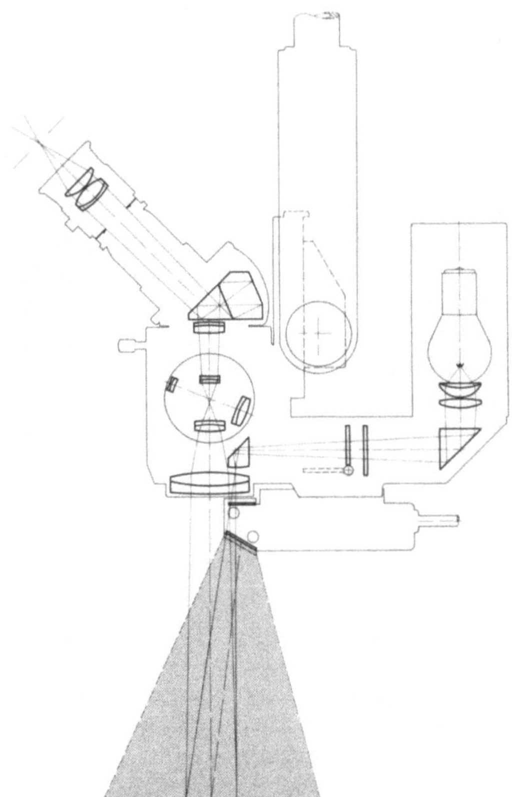

Fig. 63. Schematic side view of the illumination beam path of the electronic flash unit.

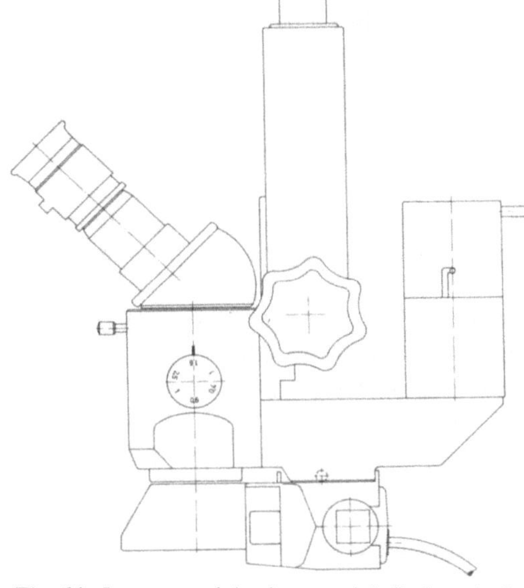

Fig. 64. Latest model of a coaxial flash unit for operation microscopes.

conditions if the demands are not critical. The most frequently used units are described below.

Fig. 62 is the side view of an operation microscope with coaxial illumination (Opmi 1) with electronic flash unit below the microscope body. Dovetails on the microscope body accept the flash which is plugged in and secured.

The schematic beam path (Fig. 63) reveals why the efficiency is unsatisfactory even if the flash output is high: due to the long working distance of operation microscope objectives from 175 mm to 400 mm focal length the illuminated field considerably exceeds the actual operating field, and the full flash energy is therefore not utilized for the latter. Compared with older types the

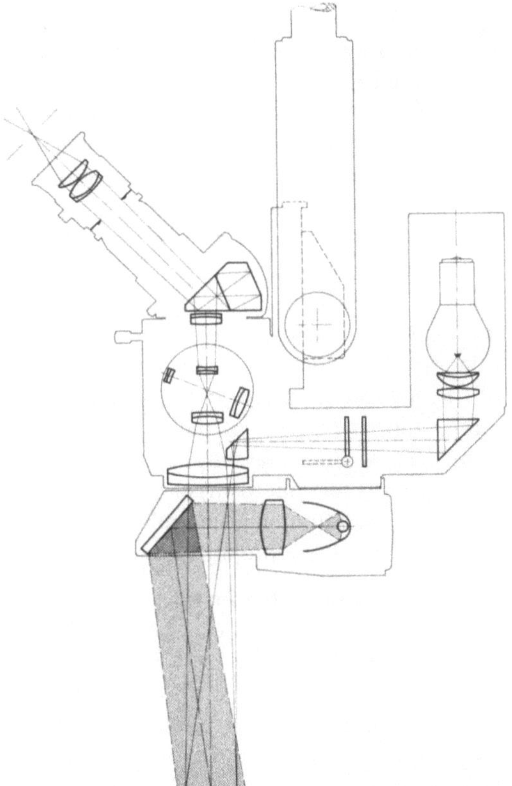

Fig. 65. Schematic side view of the new coaxial flash illuminator.

luminous efficacy of this system has been considerably increased by a lamp condenser in the latest model of a coaxial electronic flash unit (Fig. 64). The 120 or 240 Ws supply of the new flash meet all requirements even if photography is difficult.

According to Fig. 65 the new electronic flash is a coaxial system: a plane deflecting mirror relays the light bundled by the lamp condenser to the operating field. Actually the tilt of the deflecting mirror would have to be changed for every frequently used objective focal length, but the gain would not justify the expenditure, because despite the lamp condenser the illuminated field is quite large. The working distance of the new flash unit is 43 mm shorter, which is 12 mm more than that of the older model.

3.3.3 Separate oblique illuminator

For microsurgery of the anterior segments the operating field must be directionally illuminated under a large observation angle, because of the strong, direct reflections by the cornea. This called for homogeneous and slit illuminators soon after introduction of operation microscopes for ophthalmic microsurgery. Homogeneous and slit illuminator are only touched upon; details see para. 3.2.1c in connection with the built-in illumination systems. Two further illumination systems which are used independently of the operation microscope are the twin lamp and the Original Hanau operating lamps. These light sources are not specifically intended for microsurgery proper, but they serve to illuminate extended operating fields. We will therefore only glance at them.

a) Homogeneous illuminator. It is always used with the slit illuminator, because survey illumination alone does not reveal details when screening restricted areas of the cornea. The homogeneous illuminator lends itself to surveys of the entire corneal surface. With a primary objective of 175 mm focal length the illuminator produces a homogen-

eously illuminated field of 45 mm diameter. It is inclined at an angle of 27° from the microscope axis. Homogeneous and slit illuminator are shown in Fig. 45.

b) Slit illuminator. Here are again the most important data of this oblique illuminator (see also Fig. 45 and para. 3.2.1c). The slit illuminator can be turned around the (vertical) axis of the microscope and is inclined at an angle of 27° from the microscope axis with the 175 mm primary objective. The slit width illumination covers a 20 mm dia. circular field between 0 and full aperture. An adapter allows ± 10 mm transverse adjustment of the slit image.

c) 30° motorized slit lamp. In contra to the above-mentioned slit illuminator it can be turned around a horizontal axis (perpendicular to the microscope axis). For the first time pre- and post-operative biomicroscopy is possible while the patient is still on the operating table; in keratoplasty, for instance, an applied suture can be controlled during and after the surgical procedure. The lamp is attached to the microscope body by means of dovetails for easy removal and fitting.

The 30° motorized slit lamp is not meant to replace the previous slit illuminators. It is primarily intended for work with the contact lens in vitreous surgery. For this kind of work the slit must be precisely adjustable without needing the hands. The slit illuminator must move on an arc to avoid time-consuming re-focusing of the entire system, and the slit must be rotatable through at least 180°. In all these cases the axis of the incident light is limited to a narrow cone whose upper end corresponds to the operating field set. The axis of the slit lamp mentioned under b) coincides with the lateral area of the cone. Only with the adapter for ± 10 mm transverse shift from the center position does it resemble the 30° motorized slit lamp.

d) Twin lamp. The twin lamp (Fig. 66) illuminates operating fields uniformly and in-

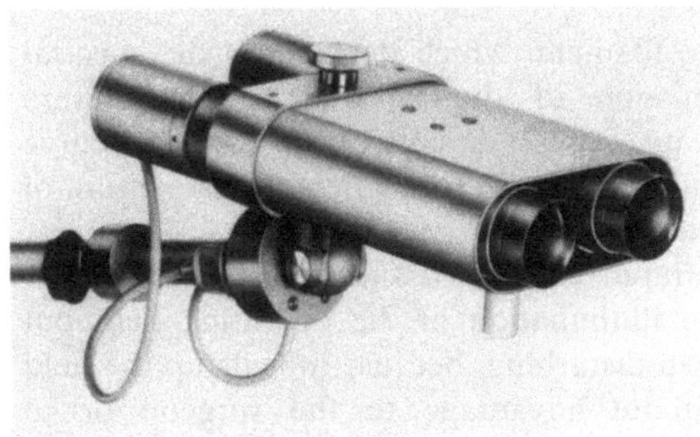

Fig. 66. Twin lamp for high-intensity illumination of narrow fields, also suitable or even required to illuminate the surrounding field in microsurgery.

tensively not for microsurgery but, for instance, for preparations without interfering with the operating team. The lamp is suspended from a separate stand, and connected with the microscope stand by means of a long double arm. The twin lamp comprises in a common housing two separate, jointly focusable illuminators. At a distance of 0.50 m the two lamps produce a homogeneous luminous field of 50 mm diameter and 30,000 lux irradiance at 6.2 V rated voltage. The irradiance increases to 40,000 lux if the lamp is run at overvoltage (6.8 V).

e) Operating lamps. The Hanaulux operating lamps are mentioned here, because they are increasingly used, especially on ceiling mounts to illuminate the operating field. They need not be suspended from a separate ceiling mount, but attach to the operation microscope's ceiling mount in optimum working position. Like microscope and accessories they are easily swung back when not needed. Technical data according to the manufacturer: Special lamp: irradiance at 44 cm distance approx. 20,000 lux; diameter of the luminous field 7 to 12 cm; Universal lamp: irradiance at a distance of 1 m 20,000 lux, diameter of the luminous field 18 cm; lamp type "London": irradiance at a distance of 1 m approx. 50,000 lux, diameter of the luminous field 22 cm. Fig. 67 shows the lamp types mentioned above on an electro-mechanical ceiling mount. The type "Hamburg" is mounted to the left, the type "London" to the right.

3.4 Filters in the illumination beam path

Filters are necessary whenever the spectral intensity distribution of the light source is not adequate for a specific application. A suitable filter changes the spectral intensity distribution, provided the unavoidable light loss it causes does not reduce the intensity in

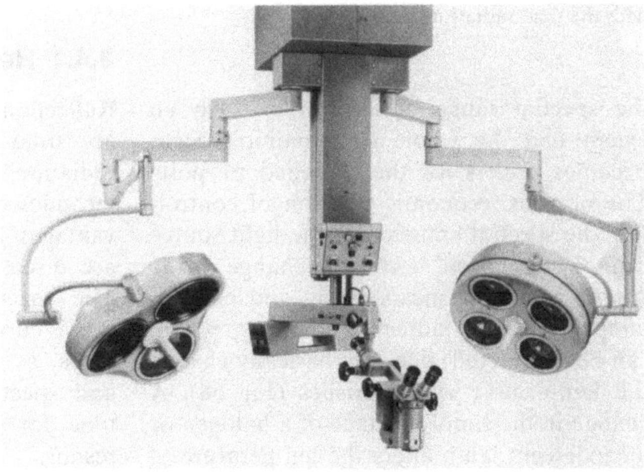

Fig. 67. Operating lamps type "Hamburg" (left) and "London" (right) on electro-mechanical ceiling mount.

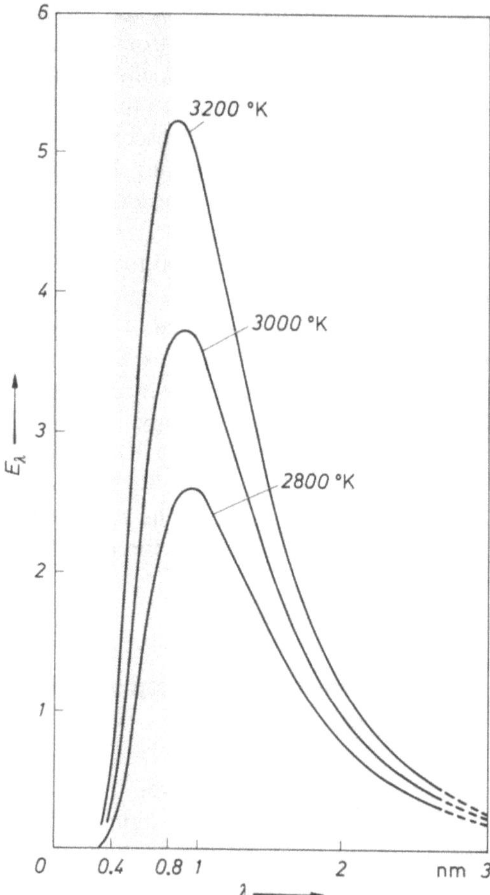

Fig. 68. Spectral emission of incandescent lamps at different temperatures (conditions are similar for halogen lamps). Note the low percentage of emission in the visible spectral range compared with the total radiation.

the spectral range of interest to such an extent that the whole illumination system becomes useless for the intended purpose. The obvious, economic solution of controlling the spectral emission of the light source cannot be realized, because a change in the supply voltage of incandescent and halogen lamps (the only adjusting parameter that can be considered) does not basically change the lamp curve characteristics (Fig. 68). A change in the supply voltage of a halogen or incandescent lamp alters the temperature of the filament, which determines the spectral emission of the lamp. The temperature change causes a shift of the emission curve and at the same time alters the maximum of the curve.

Infrared emission is not only irrelevant for the illumination of the operating field but even disturbing, because it heats up the field without advantage to the surgeon or to documentation equipment. It is the manufacturer's task to suppress the disturbing infrared light as far as possible (limits will be discussed later), which can be achieved by means of heat filters.

Contrast enhancement of the microscopic image is wanted or required in ophthalmic microsurgery, for instance. It is achieved by color glass filters (generally red-free, i.e. green filters). But the above-mentioned limit is soon reached. Another considerable portion of the small visible range emitted by the lamp must be cut off. Furthermore, the filter itself causes high losses in its own spectral range (here the green range). Though originally quite simple the problem can only be solved by a compromise.

The comprehensive introduction to the chapter about filters is meant to familiarize the microscope user with the instrument makers' difficulties in reaching such a compromise.

3.4.1 Heat filters

Reflection and absorption-type heat filters are used to filter the unwanted infrared radiation out of the wide spectral range of incandescent or halogen lamps. The advantages and disadvantages of both types are discussed in the following paragraphs. The spectral transmittance and/or reflectance curves of frequently used filters are given, as well as the product of filter curve and spectral emission curve of one lamp type for a survey of technically feasible results.

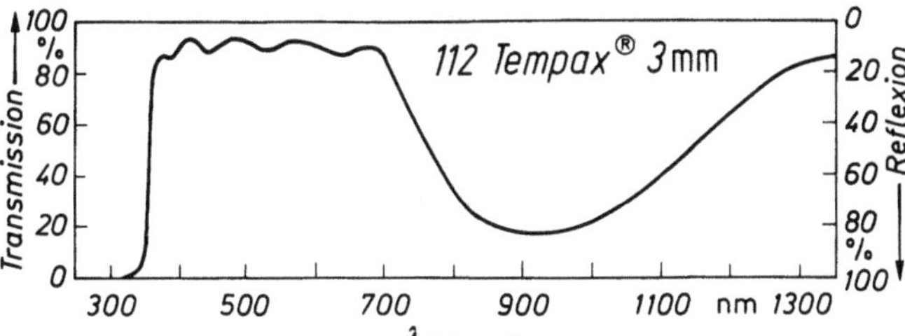

Fig. 69. Spectral transmittance curve of a reflection-type heat filter of the type 112 (e) Tempax® 3 mm. This filter does not completely suppress the infrared portion of the light but reduces it considerably.

a) Reflection-type heat filters. Their technical principle has been explained in connection with halogen lamps. The infrared radiation is filtered out from the light these lamps emit by reflection, and only the interesting, visible spectral range is radiated forward. Reflection-type heat filters follow the same principle: the disturbing infrared radiation is reflected back to the lamp, and only the visible-light rays pass through. Reflection-type heat filters do not heat up like absorption-type filters, but they require more technical outlay and are therefore more expensive. If the demands on the filtering of infrared light are high, reflection-type heat filters alone are often not efficient enough.

Fig. 69 shows the spectral transmittance curve of a reflection-type heat filter, type 112 Tempax® 3 mm, with maximum efficiency between 870 and 950 nm. In this spectral region the filter reflects approx. 80% of the incident radiation and allows only about 20% to pass through.

The interaction of heat filter and light source emission is more instructive and actually the only decisive parameter. Even if a filter has a low transmittance at a specific wavelength, the efficiency of the light source-filter combination depends in the last analysis on how low or high the light intensity of the lamp at this point. The only decisive factor is the product of the two curves (at every wavelength within the spectral range of interest), the spectral emission of the light source, and the spectral reflectance or transmittance of

the heat filter. Fig. 70 shows this product as a function of the wavelength for a combination of 30 W incandescent lamp (at rated voltage) and 112 Tempax® 3 mm heat filter. These statements reveal the following drawbacks of the above-mentioned light source-filter combination: In the visible range the curve is basically determined by the lamp emission, i.e. the intensity increases at first, towards longer wavelengths. Above 700 nm the curve drops sharply, with a minimum value at about 900 nm caused by the filter characteristics. After that there is another rise as a result of the increase of the emission curve and the greater transmission of the filter.

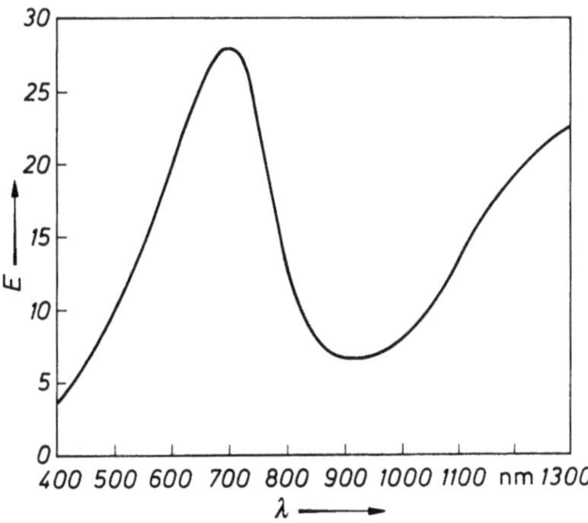

Fig. 70. Spectral curve of a 6 V 30 W incandescent lamp with reflection-type heat filter 112 Tempax® 3 mm.

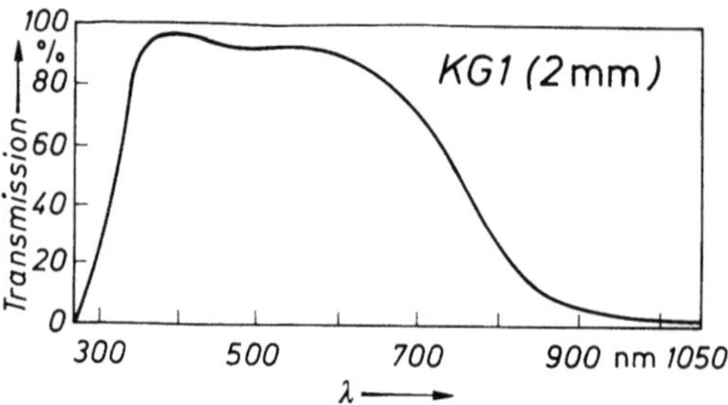

Fig. 71. Spectral transmittance curve of an absorption-type heat filter KG 1 (2 mm).

b) Absorption-type heat filters. As explained by its designation it absorbs infrared radiation, which heats it up. The heat of high-intensity light sources – even of the 6 V 30 W lamp – may eventually destroy the filter, because the absorbed radiation can only be emitted by radiation (a minute portion thereof) or conductivity, which is the only effective method. The instrument manufacturer must therefore provide effective transition of conductivity from the filter edge to the housing of the illumination beam path.

Fig. 71 shows the spectral transmittance curve of the filter. The transmission is more than 90% between 400 and 600 nm. It

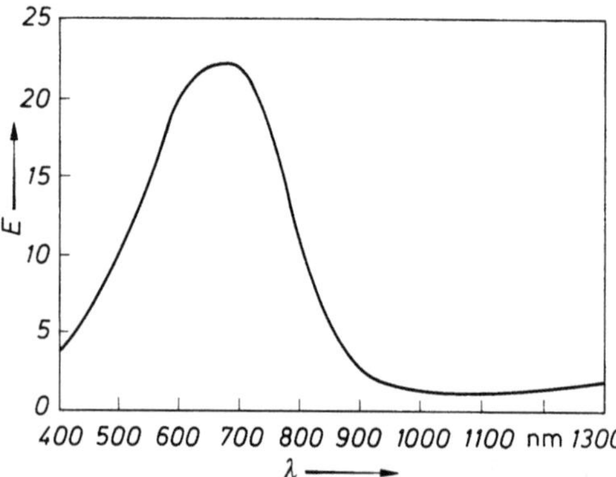

Fig. 72. Spectral intensity distribution of a 6 V 30 W incandescent lamp at rated voltage after passage of an absorption-type heat filter KG 1 (2 mm).

decreases to 70% at 700 nm, and drops to less than 10% beyond 875 nm towards the longer wavelengths, which means that the absorption exceeds 90%. Interaction with the light source is of decisive importance also for these filters. For purposes of comparison Fig. 72 shows the same type of light source (6 V 30 W) at rated load in combination with the filter type KG 1, 2 mm thick. At 1000 nm, for instance, as much as 6% of the maximum intensity at 700 nm is transmitted and can reach the operating field if the losses due to reflection and absorption in the illumination beam path behind the filter are disregarded because they are too small.

3.4.2 Color filters

Color filters are problematic only in one respect: they further reduce the low intensity of available light sources for operation microscopes in the visible range, because they reduce the maximum transmission of the narrow region of the useful visible range. Regarding the filter passband, i.e. the two slopes of the filter curve, the demands on these filters are not critical, as opposed to the high requirements for a light source-filter combination for fluorescence angiography of the fundus, where the spectral ranges of fluorescence excitation and emission must be considered for exciter and barrier filters.

a) Green filters. The contrast-enhancing filter which is most frequently used in operation microscopes is a green filter of the type Vg 6 or VG 9, each 2 mm thick. The filter curves are shown in Fig. 73. Which of the two is preferred for a specific contrast enhancement cannot be objectively decided because due to the physical color hue the choice depends on the surgeon's subjective impression. The curve of a light source/green filter combination is therefore not shown.

b) Blue filters (cobalt filter). The considerations with respect to the green filter also

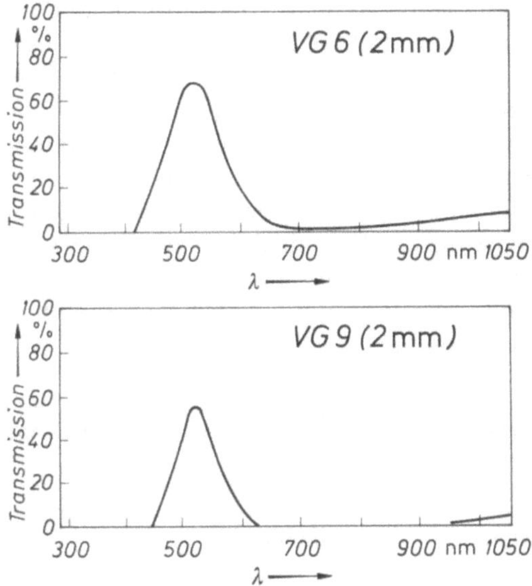

Fig. 73. Spectral transmittance curves of the green filters VG 6 and VG 9, each 2 mm thick.

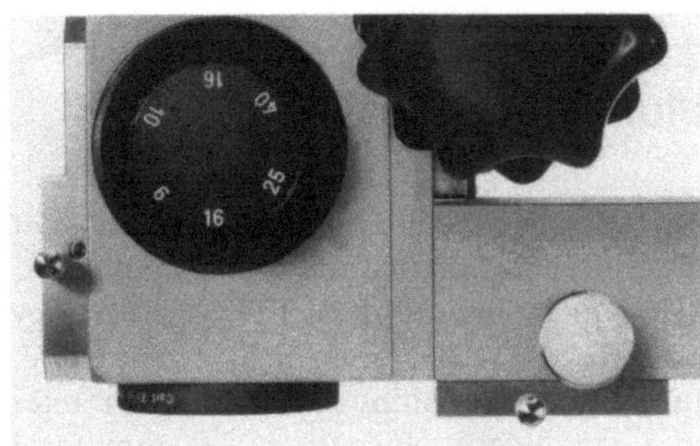

Fig. 75. Knurled knob on operation microscope Opmi 1 which swings a green filter into the illumination beam path.

apply to the blue filter BG 12 for contrast enhancement of the image in an operation microscope. It is not described in detail because it is less frequently used than the green filter. Fig. 74 shows the spectral transmittance curve of the 2 mm thick filter BG 12. Like the green filter its slopes are not steep, i.e. not critical. However, the filter transmits only 79% of the incident radiation. Its practical use is limited by the reduced effective intensity of blue light.

c) Insertion of filters in the beam path. The insertion of filters in the illumination beam path does not concern heat filters which are integral with the beam path. Color filters are needed only occasionally and are quickly swung in by means of a knurled knob on the side wall of the microscope body containing the illumination beam path (Fig. 75) of the operation microscopes Opmi 1, 6, and 9. Since there is no need for one and the same medical discipline to interchange rapidly between a green and a blue filter, only one of the two is inserted.

The new operation microscopes of the type Opmi 1 H and 6 H are equipped with a filter slider (Fig. 76) which is readily taken out, e.g. for filter exchange. The two green filters VG 6 and VG 9 also fit in the slider for insertion in the beam path.

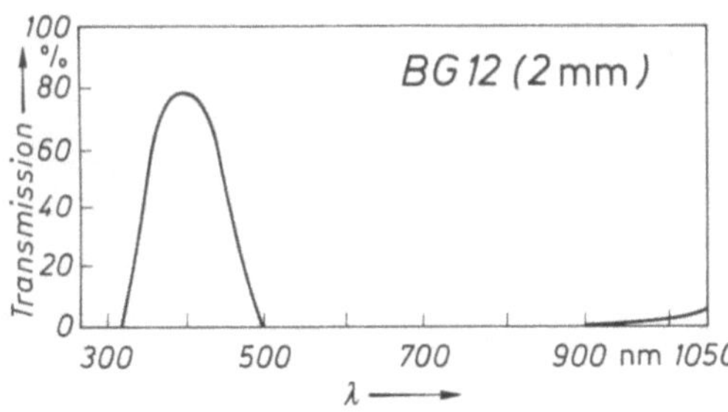

Fig. 74. Transmittance curve of a blue filter (also known as cobalt filter) BG 12 (2 mm thick).

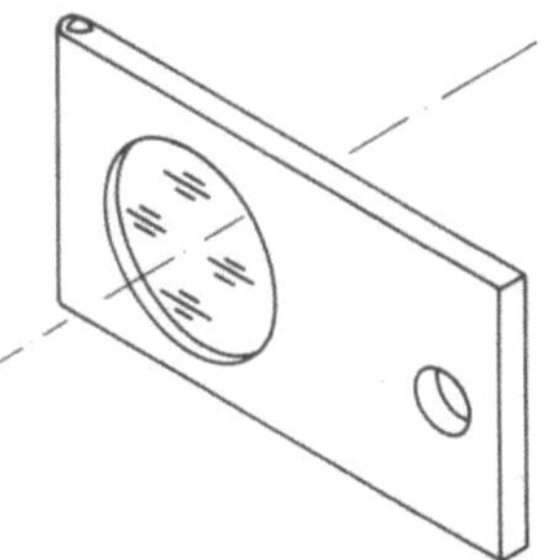

Fig. 76. Filter slider of operation microscopes Opmi 1 H and Opmi 6 H.

3.5 Comparison of different illumination systems

The following Tables 6 to 9 give a survey of the different illumination systems described in the foregoing chapters. The intensity they produce in the operating field is compared. Intensity and luminous-field diameter refer to a microscope objective of 200 mm focal length. This is permissible for all coaxial illumination systems, and for oblique illuminators, but not for the 30° motorized slit lamp, where because of the arc the values refer to the 175 mm objective. This rule cannot be adhered to for separate illuminators, or for Hanau operating lamps, although they are connected with the microscope stand. Due to the unavoidable scattering of all lamp data the indicated intensities are only approximate values with a deviation of max. ± 15%.

Table 6. Coaxial illumination systems
Comparison of different illumination systems. Main objective $f_O = 200$ mm

Microscope	Source	Illumination
Opmi 6 S	6 V 30 W	22,000 lux = 2,040 footcandles
Opmi 6 F	12 V 100 W	30,000 lux = 2,790 footcandles
Opmi 6 H	12 V 100 W	160,000 lux = 14,860 footcandles

Table 7. Oblique illuminators *on* the microscope
Comparison of different illumination systems. Main objective $f_O = 200$ mm

Type	Illumination
Focusable illuminator	9,000 lux = 840 footcandles
Fiber optics for oblique illumination	32,000 lux = 2,970 footcandles

Table 8. Oblique illuminators *connected* with the microscope
Comparison of different illumination systems

Type	Illumination
Homogeneous illuminator	17,000 lux = 1,580 footcandles
Slit illuminator	9,000 lux = 840 footcandles
30° motorized slit illuminator (halogen bulb)	10,000 lux = 930 footcandles

Table 9. *Separate* oblique illuminators
Comparison of different illumination systems

Type	Illumination
Twin lamp (0.5 m distance)	30,000 lux = 2,790 footcandles
Operating lamps (1.0 m distance)	
Type "Universal"	20,000 lux = 1,860 footcandles
"London"	50,000 lux = 4,650 footcandles

4 Couplings

An operation microscope and its accessories can be brought into a certain position for a specific application by a choice of different couplings. No operation microscope in whatever field of application can remain in one and the same position during a surgical procedure, but must be adjusted to different working positions which depend on the medical discipline and the kind of operation. This applies in particular to ear, nose, throat (ENT) and neurosurgery, where an operation microscope must be quickly and easily brought into the "correct" working position without much ado and effort. To achieve this, the microscope must

a) be coarsely adjustable in height, in depth and sideways, which is realized by carrier arms (and accessories). Details see chapter 5;

b) at least be rotatable around one axis, sometimes even around three axes, and capable of axial focusing.

These requirements which are of great importance for the different microsurgical procedures call for a number of couplings, which are explained below in connection with the microscopes. To avoid repetition the basic equipment in a wider sense – type of illumination and stand, for instance – will be described. A list of available couplings will be found at the end of this section.

Some explanations beforehand. The designation "operation microscope" comprises the microscope proper and the holding "bracket" in which the microscope pivots. Fig. 77 shows the bracket of an earlier operation microscope model Opmi 1 with 5-stage magnification changer and coaxial illuminator. This holding bracket was developed and used at a time when no accessories were available for operation microscopes. But with the introduction of the beam splitter making co-observation and photography possible, operation microscopes had to be tiltable and space-saving. In spite of this the holder had to be of utmost stability. The operation microscopes Opmi 1 and 6 and the diagnosis microscope Opmi 9 (Fig. 78) were mounted on one-sided, rugged holding brackets. Double microscopes for ophthalmic microsurgery are mounted differently. The main microscope is vertical, while the second, assistant's microscope is inclined at an angle of 27° from the main microscope's axis and must be rotatable around the same vertical axis as the main microscope. The Opmi 5, which is the first double microscope after Harms [6], features 5-stage magnification changers for surgeon and assistant in

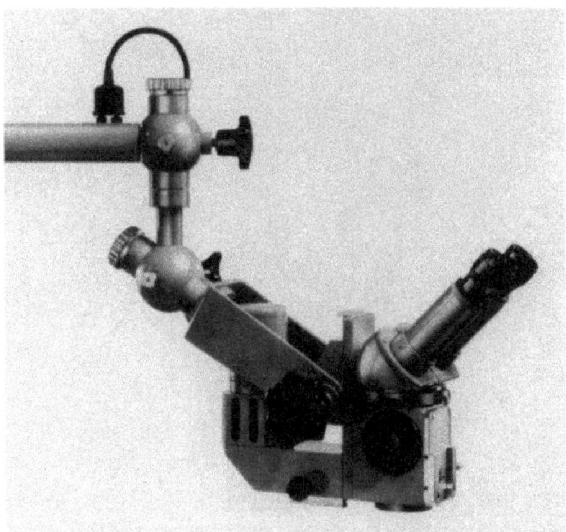

Fig. 77. Older model of operation microscope Opmi 1 with two-sided holding bracket for rotatable mounting of the microscope.

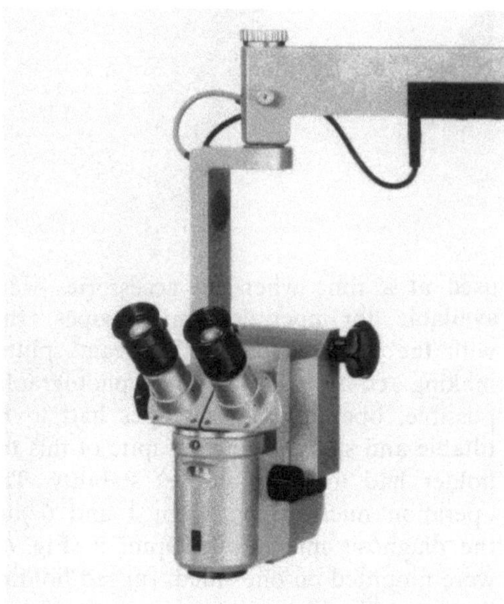

Fig. 78. Latest, one-sided holding bracket for operation microscopes Opmi 1, 6 and 9, formerly two-sided bracket.

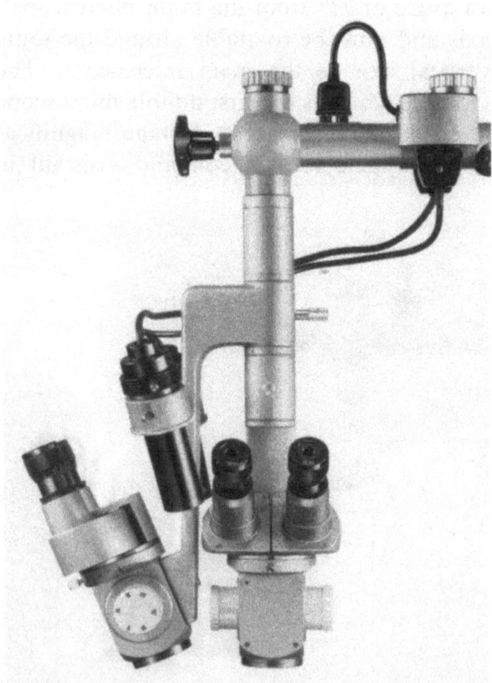

Fig. 79. Double microscope after Harms. Main and assistant's microscope can be rotated around a common vertical axis.

both microscopes (Fig. 79). The principle has been retained for a later version of the instrument, but the main microscope is now equipped with a zoom system instead of the 5-stage magnification changer. The second microscope still features the 5-stage magnification changer, because the assistant must not change magnification as often as the surgeon, provided the magnification of his microscope is, for instance, 1.25× higher than that of the main microscope. Homogeneous and slit illuminators on the Opmi 8 and the former Opmi 5 must also be rotatable around the same vertical axis, which explains the special vertical mounting of double microscopes, which differs completely from the mounting of all other microscopes. Details are given in the following chapters.

4.1 Basic equipment for different microsurgical disciplines

The different disciplines are dealt with below in alphabetical order.

4.1.1 Hand surgery

a) **Opmi 2 operation microscope.** This model is no longer manufactured, but it is described here, because instruments are still in use in many hospitals. The demands on a microscope for hand surgery have been mentioned before, and are supplemented below by special requirements, especially regarding the couplings. By means of a cardan coupling (Fig. 80) the operation microscope can be rotated around three mutually perpendicular (one vertical and two horizontal) axes. The microscope holder is one-sided so as to leave sufficient space for a stereo beam splitter and many accessories. The cardan coupling provides a third carrier arm which is required for hand surgery.
Fig. 80 shows that all electrical supply lines

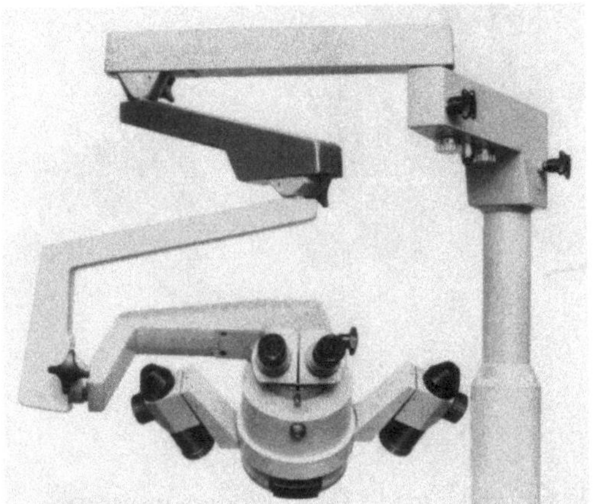

Fig. 80. Cardan coupling of older zoom microscope model Opmi 2.

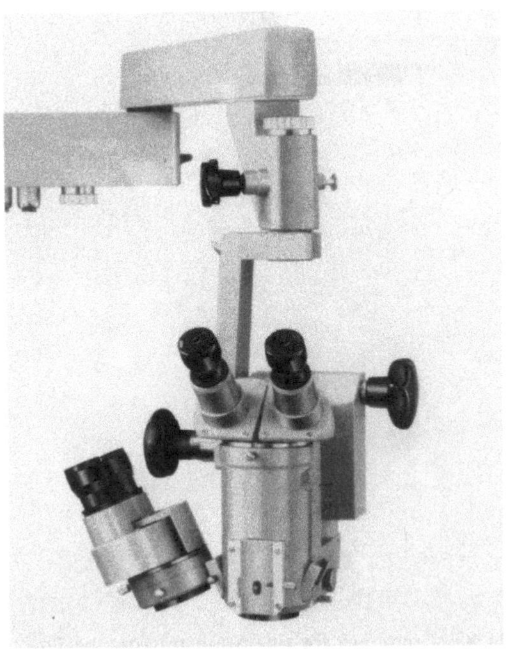

Fig. 81. Quick-change coupling with Opmi 6.

for microscope illumination, motorized zoom system and precision focusing are inside the coupling. This also applies to the quick-change coupling (Fig. 81) which is easily removed for sterilization and re-attached without need of tools. For hand surgery an $x-y$ coupling can be attached to any Opmi 2 operation microscope no matter how long it has been in use (Fig. 82) for foot- or hand-panel-controlled ± 25 mm motorized horizontal precision adjustment of the microscope.

b) Opmi 7 D operation microscope. It is equipped with a new type of coupling. According to Fig. 83 the vertical axis corresponds to that of the above instrument, but the point of rotation of the horizontal axis lies in the short coupling piece above the microscope. This limits the precision adjusting range of the microscope compared with the above-mentioned instrument, but the coupling is sufficient for practical work, because in hand surgery only minor tilting of the microscope is necessary. Therefore it is assumed that the user will accept that after tilting the microscope he has to refocus it by means of the height adjustment of the stand. (This applies to all microscopes in all disciplines. Only the way the focusing is done is different.)

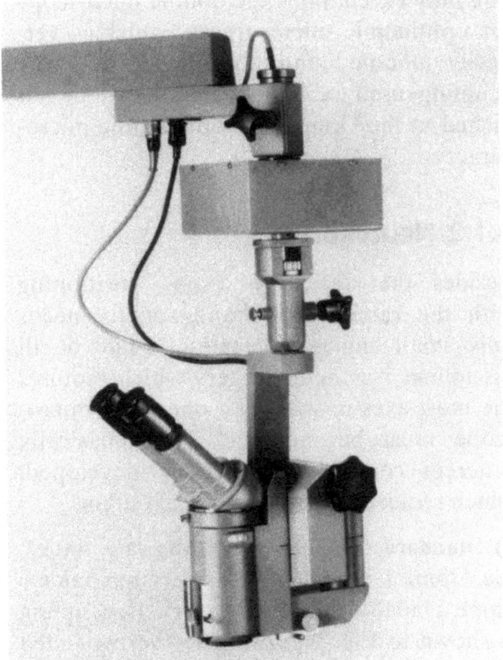

Fig. 82. Opmi 6 for hand surgery with $x-y$ coupling for motorized precision adjustment of the microscope.

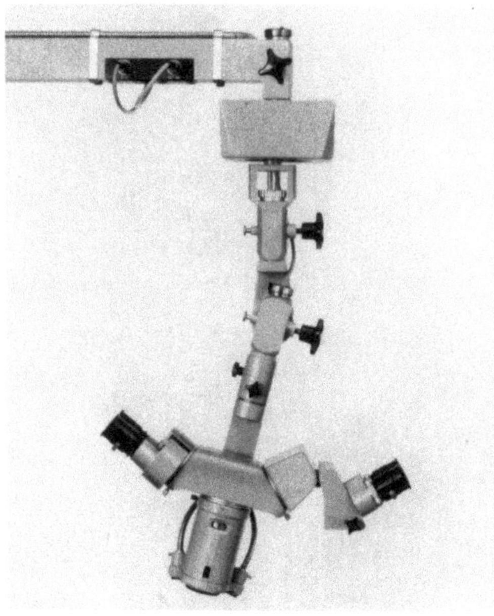

Fig. 83. Couplings for operation microscope Opmi 7 D.

The only exception is the double microscope for ophthalmic microsurgery, which is vertically mounted and not tilted. The same coupling used in hand surgery can be attached to the Opmi 3 for ophthalmic microsurgery.

4.1.2 Neurosurgery

Besides the necessary coarse positioning with the carrier arm, hand surgery needs only small angles of rotation, while of all disciplines it is neurosurgery which requires the most axes in which an operation microscope must be movable. Three basically different couplings have been developed, which require different technical outlay.

a) Standard coupling. Until the late sixties, the Opmi 1 was the only operation microscope available for neurosurgery. Its coupling is shown in Fig. 84. Owing to the two-sided mounting bracket, treatment of a seated patient is limited if the microscope is turned about the horizontal axis. Since 1970 the

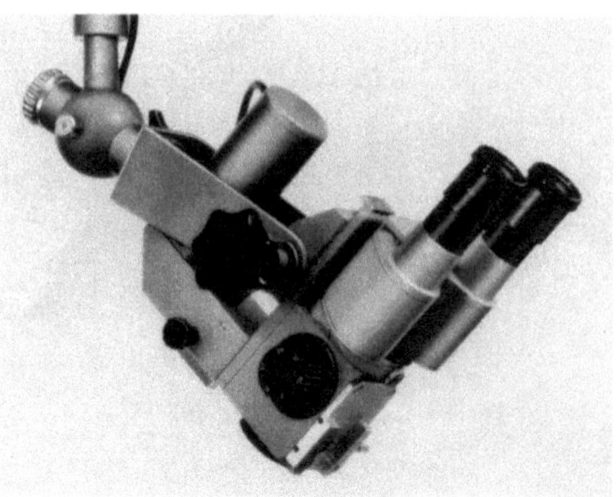

Fig. 84. Older model Opmi 1 for neurosurgery.

mounting is a one-sided bracket, also suitable for the latest microscope types 1 F and 1 H, 6 F and 6 H (Fig. 85).

b) Inclined coupling. A more universal coupling for neurosurgery introduced at about the same time as the above (Fig. 86). In addition to the features of the standard coupling it can be rotated about an axis at an angle to the operating field. If the microscope is in vertical or slightly deviating working position, this coupling leaves much more space for accessories above the microscope body. The inclined coupling can also be attached to all operation microscopes of the type 1 (with 5-stage Galilean magnifica-

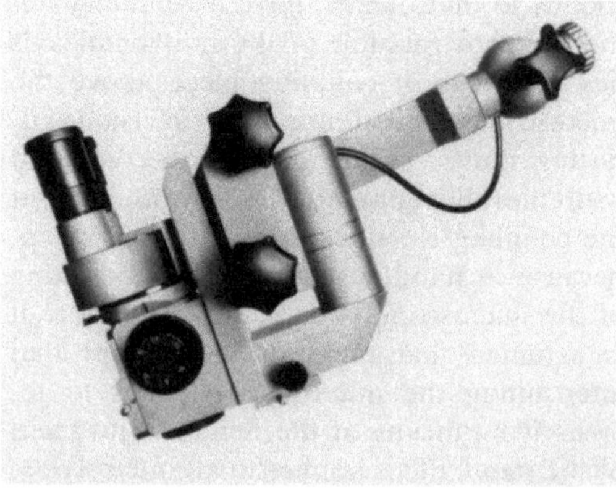

Fig. 85. Opmi 1 S for neurosurgery on one-sided bracket.

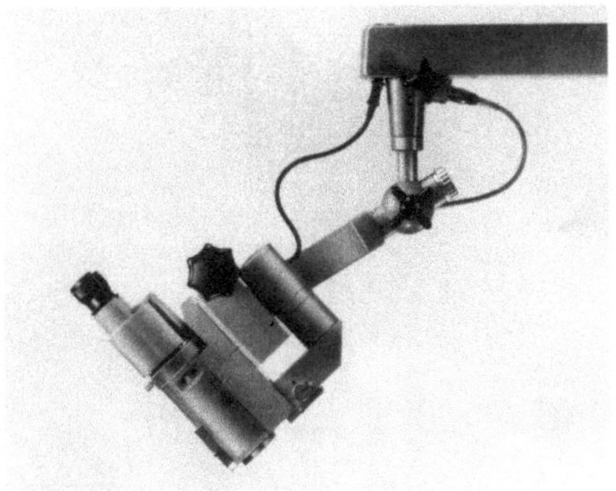

Fig. 86. Opmi 6 on inclined coupling.

tion changer, including the types 1 F and 1 H) and 6 (zoom microscope, including the types 6 F and 6 H).

c) Mobile coupling. This mounting (Fig. 87) which is now some years old differs essentially from the above-mentioned suspensions and couplings of microscopes for neurosurgery. With the aid of this ingenious, sophisticated system the operation microscope is easily and quickly brought into any desired position for neurosurgical procedures, because the microscope can be tilted about three mutually perpendicular axes and in addition adjusted in the three spatial coordinates. The adjustment is electrically controlled, and if the control is interrupted, electromagnetic clutches secure the adjusted position. The function can be taken over by two switches: coarse adjustment is done with switches in the handles on either side of the microscope, but the Yaşargil operation microscope with the mounting he initiated can only be effectively utilized with the mouth switch (Fig. 88). The design is based on the following idea.

Cerebral operations, the removal of a microaneurysm, for instance, must be made at high microscope magnification, which in turn limits the microscope's depth of focus. If microinstruments are introduced into the operating field the tissue yields owing to its

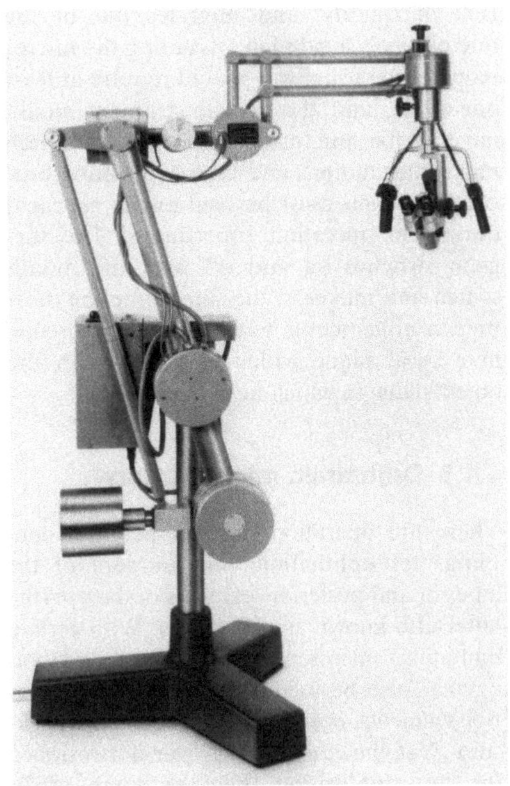

Fig. 87. Opmi 1 suspended from a special mobile coupling which allows adjustment in six different axes.

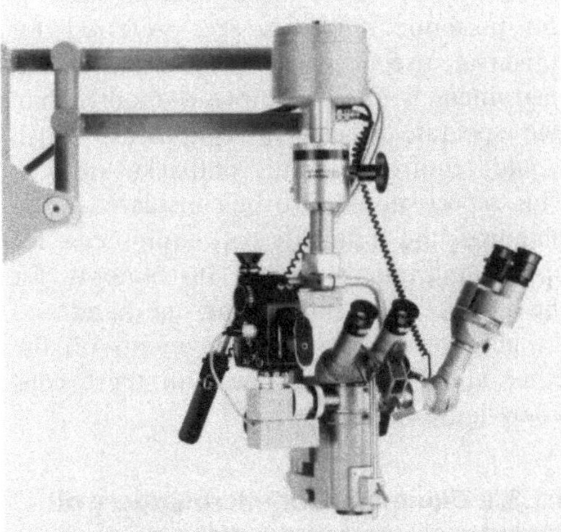

Fig. 88. Mouth switch (beneath the binocular tube) which releases the electro-magnetic lock of the microscope adjustment.

lack of rigidity, and migrates out of the microscope's focal plane. Guiding the microscope in the usual way would require at least one hand, and the microinstrument would have to be put aside. The mouth switch makes this tedious and time-consuming procedure, which must be continually repeated during an operation superfluous. The surgeon switches on and off with the mouth switch and makes at the same time the most precise adjustments to keep the microscope in a focal plane which coincides with the object plane in which he is working.

4.1.3 Opthalmic microsurgery

There are operation microscopes and couplings for ophthalmic microsurgery of the anterior and posterior segments of the eye (the latter also known as retinology). With certain limitations microscope equipment for retinology can also be used for surgery of the anterior segments, because it has all necessary features. Yet, the equipment is over-dimensioned for this application, because some of its functions are not needed while others which create ideal conditions for surgery of the anterior segments of the eye are lacking. Despite such shortcomings instruments for the posterior segments are preferred for universal use, because one sophisticated instrument is after all more economic than two separate pieces of equipment, which would require economic cutbacks anyway. This aspect should also be considered when planning the purchase of equipment for ophthalmic microsurgery. Instruments for the anterior segments on the one hand and for anterior and posterior segments on the other are discussed below with these considerations in mind.

4.1.3.1 Equipment for microsurgery of the anterior segments of the eye

a) Straight coupling. The mounting of Opmi 3, the operation microscope developed for

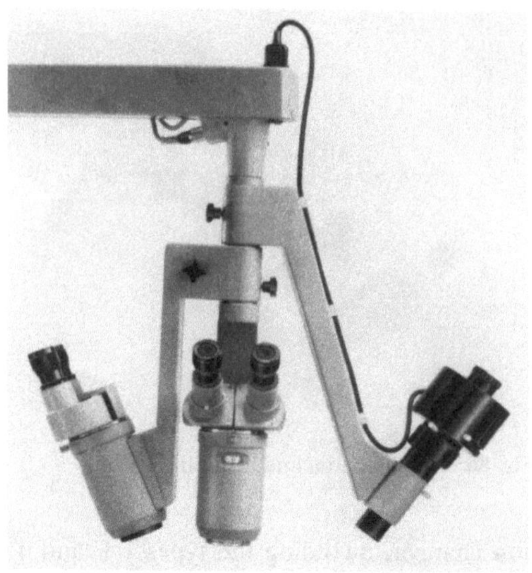

Fig. 89. Mounting for operation microscopes Opmi 3, 5 and 8.

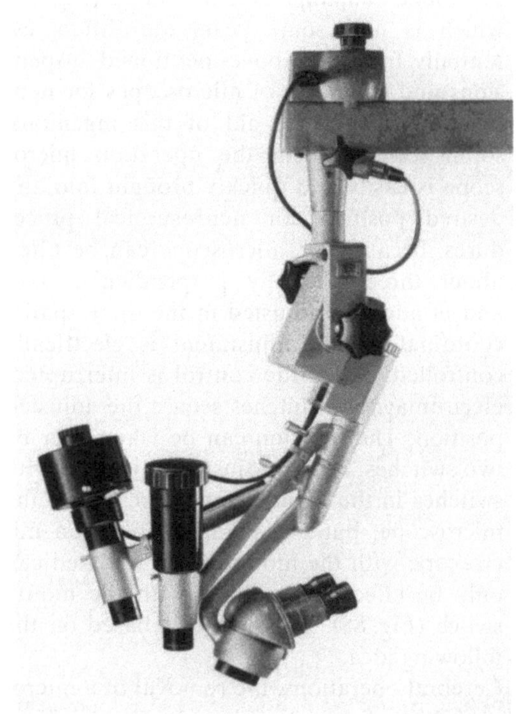

Fig. 90. Coupling for Opmi 3 to adjust minor tilts of the microscope from the vertical axis. A simple inclined coupling as shown in Fig. 86 without axial focusing and without rack and pinion for instrument tilt can also be used.

and named after Barraquer, anticipated the mountings of all following models. This applies not only to the Barraquer cine microscope (Opmi 4), but also to the Harms double microscopes (Opmi 5 with 5-stage magnification changer) and the latest model Opmi 8 with zoom systems [9 f]. The features particulary in question here are the mounting and the rotation of the microscope (and of the illuminators which are less important in this respect) around the vertical axis (Fig. 89).

b) Tilt coupling. A coupling for minor tilting of the microscope (Fig. 90), exclusively for operation microscopes Opmi 3. The microscope is preferably used in tilted position, for turning it on a cone surface to inspect sutures, for instance after cataract extraction or cornea transplantations.

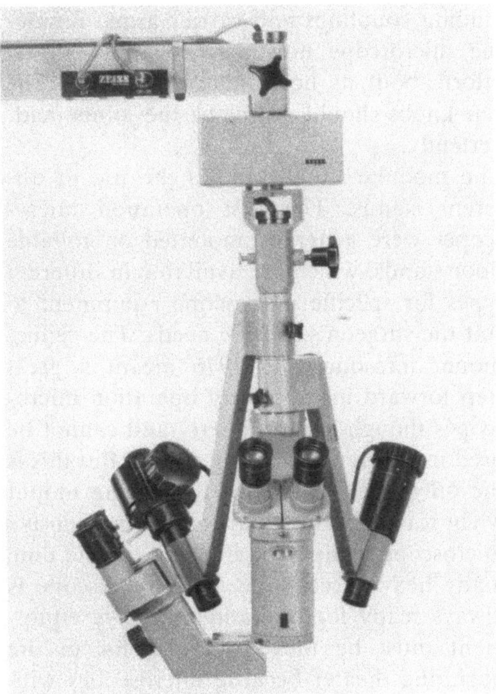

Fig. 91. $x - y$ coupling for motorized precision adjustment of the zoom microscope Opmi 7 in two coordinates, here with slit and homogeneous illuminator and 8° assistant's microscope.

c) $x - y$ **coupling.** A coupling that has been on the market for some years already. It is used together with the straight and tilt couplings (paras. a) and b)), for more comfortable working and time-saving surgical procedures (Fig. 91). Hand- or foot-panel-controlled the microscope's adjusting range is ± 25 mm, at a speed of approx. 5 mm/s.

4.1.3.2 Equipment for microsurgery of anterior and posterior segments of the eye

With some restrictions these are the more "universal" microscopes, for the anterior and posterior segments of the eye, primarily because of their coaxial illuminators. Those particulary concerned are the microscope models 1 and 1 F with 5-stage magnification changer, the zoom microscopes 6 and 6 F and last but not least the latest zoom microscope model 7 F. Except for the last one all microscopes feature an axial focusing facility which is manually controlled in the types 1 and 1 F and hand- or foot-panel-controlled. in the older zoom microscopes 6 and 6 F; the latest models offer the option of manual or motorized axial focusing. The microscopes Opmi 6 and 6 F can in addition be tilted about a horizontal axis by means of a gear-controlled tilt system with which the microscope can be positioned even for most sophisticated and complex surgical procedures.

One piece of microscope equipment for microsurgery of the anterior and posterior segments of the eye shall serve as an example (Fig. 92). All microscopes for retinological microsurgery must fulfill one important condition: motorized positioning of microscope and comprehensive, heavy accessories because of the narrow geometrical conditions, for instance, in vitreous surgery, which can only be achieved with the above-mentioned $x - y$ coupling.

Another requirement in vitreous surgery, for instance, is the motorized 30° slit lamp, which is available for the microscopes 1

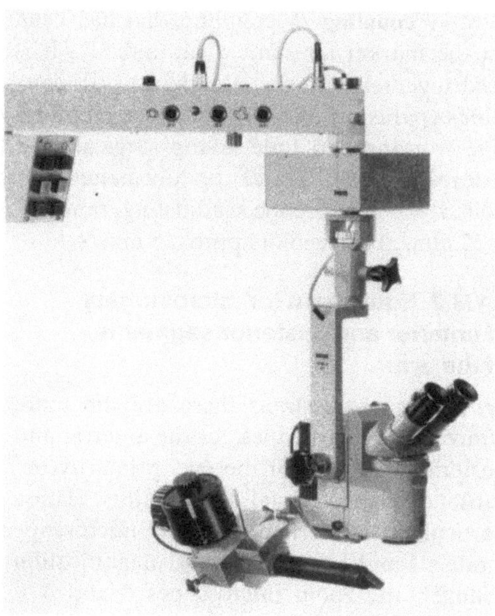

Fig. 92. Opmi 6 S with ± 30° operation slit illuminator and $x-y$ coupling on electro-mechanical ceiling mount.

(with manual magnification changer) and the zoom microscopes 6. It is easily attached (also subsequently) to both microscope types and removed when not needed.

4.1.4 Otorhinolaryngology

In the course of time standard equipment has developed for otoscopic and laryngoscopic microsurgery. Operation microscopes with 5-stage magnification changer are the most frequently used. Zoom microscopes have recently gained increasing popularity owing to foot-panel-controlled magnification change and full-size magnification for documentation. They also allow non-manual rapid change from low-power magnification for a survey of the operating field to high-power magnification of features, e.g. for stapes surgery.

Operation microscopes used in operating theaters are discussed below classified according to the illumination system, not the frequency of their use or applicability. Owing to the modular system one and the same stand accepts different microscope models, couplings and carrier arms. One piece of equipment representative of all the others is described in each of the following paragraphs.

All operation microscopes for otorhinolaryngology have coaxial illumination systems in common (para. 3.3.1), of different types, of course, and with different light sources. All microscopes feature swing-in green filters. Only operation microscopes with built-in 12 V 100 W halogen lamp have an iris diaphragm in the illumination beam path to vary the size of the field of view continuously from 32 mm to approx. 4 mm diameter.

Last but not least the microscope must be of extraordinary maneuverability, ensured by counterweights in the stand which balance the weight of microscope and accessories, including couplings and carrier arms. Besides the microscope must be movable without effort about its horizontal or tilt axis. The star knobs should not block the joints inadvertently.

The modular design allows the use of different stands. The first operation microscopes were generally mounted on rollable floor stands, which are available in different types for specific microscope equipment to suit the surgeon's specific needs. The ceiling mount introduced in 1976 meant a great step forward in the use of operation microscopes though it is stationary and cannot be used in different operating rooms. But this is the only disadvantage of the ceiling mount when it is desirable to attach comprehensive microscope equipment and at the same time many heavy accessories. The microscope is always ready for use, and no heavy equipment must be moved to and for in the operating theater because microscopes with heavy accessories must for reasons of stability be mounted on equally heavy stands.

a) Operation microscopes Opmi 1, 6, and 6 S. Fig. 93 shows an operation microscope

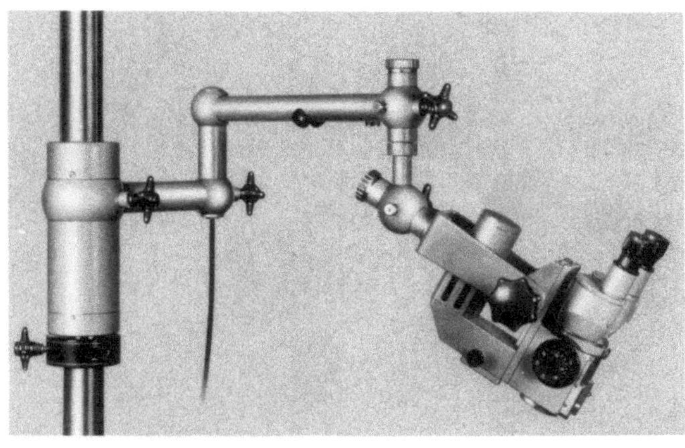

Fig. 93. Operation microscope Opmi 1 with two carrier arms, inclined coupling and 5-stage magnification changer, with integral coaxial illumination system.

Opmi 1 with 5-stage magnification changer, the longest in use of the operation microscopes. It is equally well suited for otoscopic and laryngoscopic surgery. A third carrier arm forms with the others a "Wullstein suspension" which adds considerably to the microscope's mobility (Fig. 94). The 30 W lamp of the microscope can be replaced by a 50 W lamp, for instance, for still or cine photography or for co-observation. Besides microscopes with 5-stage magnification changer instruments of the same optical quality but with zoom magnification system have been available for some years, first of all the older type with a zoom factor of 1:5, which was succeeded by a more compact version with a zoom range from 0.5× to 2.0×. The motorized zoom system is provided with manual override.

Operation microscopes with built-in halogen illumination systems are special developments for this kind of work.

b) Operation microscopes Opmi 1 H and 6 H. The operation microscopes Opmi 1 H and 6 H with built-in 12 V 100 W halogen lamps instead of the 30 W and 50 W incandescent lamps have also been on the market since 1976. Even at normal load the 12 V 100 W lamps supply two tims more intensity than the 50 W incandescent lamp at overload. But operation at overload drastically reduces the life of the lamp (see paras. 3.1.1 and 3.1.2). Halogen lamps are therefore particularly suited for still and cine photography. The above-mentioned microscopes are equipped with a filter slider which accepts either two green filters of different density for different contrast enhancement, or a combination of green and blue filters. The microscopes also feature an iris diaphragm for contrast enhancement by suppression of straylight. In photography, for instance, this diaphragm is used to single out a feature of the operating field from the surrounding field by illumination alone. Fig. 95 shows an operation microscope Opmi 6 H on ceiling mount with three carrier arms and inclined coupling. For laryngoscopy the

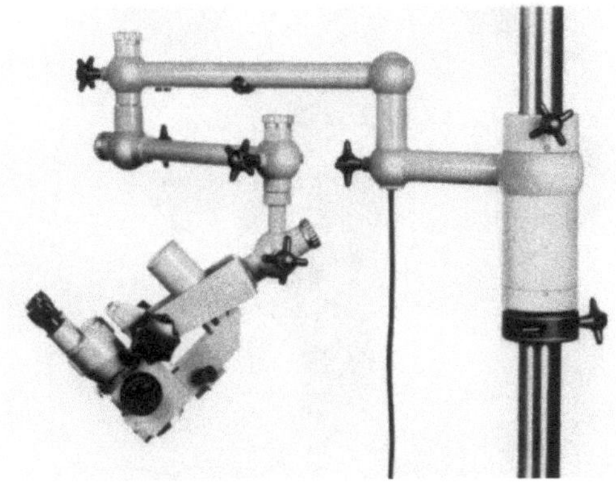

Fig. 94. Operation microscope Opmi 1 with 5-stage magnification changer on inclined coupling with three carrier arms. (Wullstein suspension)

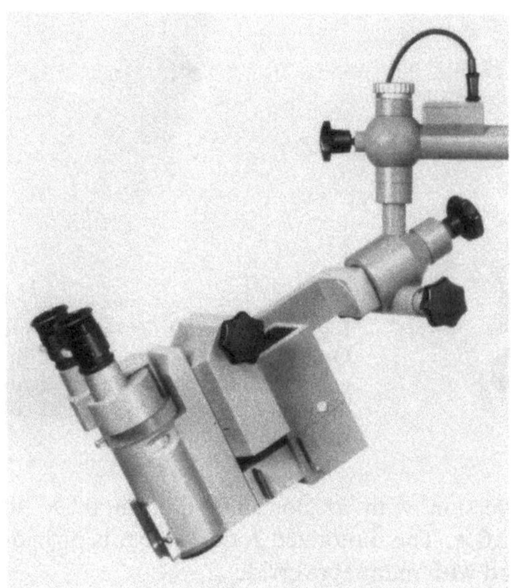

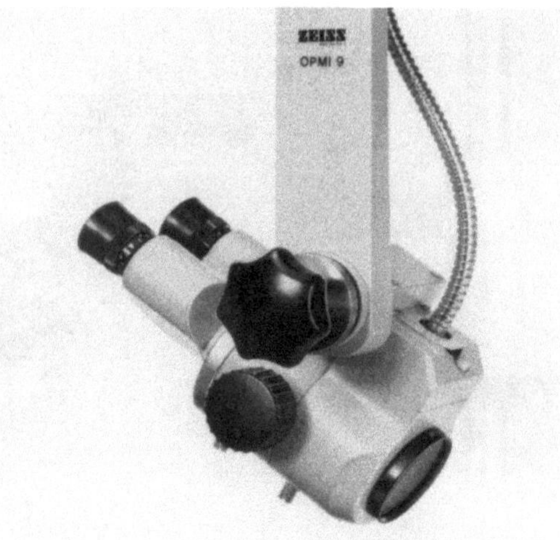

Fig. 96. Operation microscope Opmi 9 F with 3-stage magnification changer and objective focusing attachment on wall swivel arm.

Fig. 95. Operation microscope Opmi 6 H with zoom system, integral 12 V 100 W halogen lamp, mounted on an inclined coupling.

ceiling mount can be easily and quickly adjusted vertically, while the alternative manual or motorized vertical adjustment will generally be chosen for surgery of the ear.

c) Operation microscopes Opmi 9 and 9 F. Simple, handy microscopes, especially for the general practitioner or for postoperative case control, with coaxial illumination, of course. The two microscopes differ essentially in the illumination: the Opmi 9 is equipped with a 30 W incandescent lamp, the Opmi 9 F with a fiber optics illumination system. The integral fiber optics system makes the microscope's dimensions particularly favorable. Opmi 9 and 9 F can be mounted on a rollable floor stand or on a wall mount to save space. Without limitation of the microscope's functions it can also be included in an ENT diagnostic unit. Fig. 96 shows an Opmi 9 F, and Fig. 97 and Opmi 9 with additional equipment. The microscope can be subsequently fitted with a magnification changer for three different magnifica-

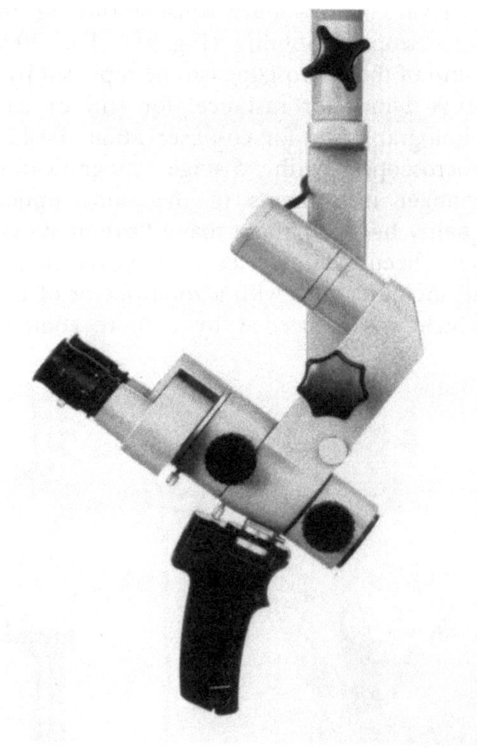

Fig. 97. Operation microscope Opmi 9 with 3-stage magnification changer, objective focusing attachment and handle.

tions. The use of a green filter is also possible. An accessory fitted to the lower part of the microscope body allows fine focusing within a range of ± 12 mm, which is quite adequate for ENT surgery.

4.1.5 Vascular and plastic surgery, and surgery of peripheral nerves

Operation microscopes with 5-stage magnification changer or zoom system are used for this kind of surgery. The first type lends itself if the budget is limited, but the different models of the zoom microscopes are especially recommended because of the foot-panel-controlled, motorized magnification change and focusing. Another important criterion is the illumination system. Coaxial illumination is always preferable, but co-observation and documentation require additional oblique illumination of the operating field. A coaxial system supplies shadow-free illumination of a small field (32 mm dia. with 200 mm objective focal length). Modern supplementary oblique illumination systems are always fiber optics systems, which can also be subsequently fitted. Besides high illumination intensity of the operating field such a system also illuminates the surrounding field (luminous field dia. approx. 75 mm with 200 mm objective focal length). Green filters are needed in vascular surgery for contrast enhancement; they are swung into the illumination beam path of all microscope types. The fact that the filters reduce the illumination intensity must be considered for the choice of the illumination system and thus the microscope, especially in view of co-observation equipment and double microscopes which are needed for plastic, vascular, and reconstructive surgery. Contrary to co-observation equipment and double microscopes, assistant's microscopes do not cause additional light losses in the surgeon's microscope.

Assistant's and double microscopes differ in the following points:

I) Double microscopes offer surgeon and assistant exactly the same viewing angle on the operating field, while assistant's microscopes are always rigidly or rotatably connected with the main microscope. Main and assistant's microscope have therefore different viewing directions on the operating field. The different instrument types are described in section 6.2.

II) The two microscopes of a double microscope configuration subtend an angle of 180°; surgeon and assistant are facing each other. A special assistant's microscope that is, however, not used in a double microscope configuration subtends an angle of 90°; in all other models this angle is variable, but in practice the optimum inclination is about 60°.

III) Another fundamental difference is the stereo beam splitter of the double microscopes (see para. 6.3.2) which brings about approx. 50% light loss for the surgeon.

IV) The operation microscope Opmi 8 D is a configuration which consists of a double microscope and an assistant's microscope.

Microscope, assistant's microscope and accessories must be tiltable for reconstructive, plastic or vascular surgery, which requires at least one coupling of the available ample selection (see illustrations in the next sections), depending on the application. Sophisticated equipment will always include an $x - y$ coupling for precision adjustment of microscope and accessories. To tilt the microscope even by small amounts, the binocular tiltable tube is recommended, which offers surgeon and assistant the choice of their viewing angle for most comfortable and relaxed working.

Rollable stands are the rule because they can be used in different operating theaters. They can be divided into two groups: Universal floor stands for support and power supply of basic equipment, with provision for power supply of documentation equipment, and extra-heavy, motorized floor stands for more sophisticated, heavier equipment. For details see chapter 5. The disadvantage of mobile stands, namely that they are difficult to position, especially with heavy equipment, is overcome by a stationary electro-mechanical ceiling mount which saves for an anaesthesist the space that is usually occupied by a floor stand with one or even two assistant's microscopes. Examples of basic equipment of operation microscopes:

a) Operation microscopes Opmi 1, 1 F, and 1 H. The simplest version shown in Fig. 98 is the Opmi 1 with 5-stage magnification changer and assistant's microscope (older type, exclusively with 27° inclination, the new one has 8° inclination). The series also includes two microscopes with different illumination systems: Opmi 1 F with coaxial illumination and fiber optics system. Compared with the Opmi 1 it is more compact and illuminates a larger field with the same intensity. Opmi 1 H comes with high-intensity 12 V 100 W light source for documentation.

b) Operation microscopes Opmi 6, 6 S, 6 F, and 6 H. This series includes microscopes with different magnification ranges of the

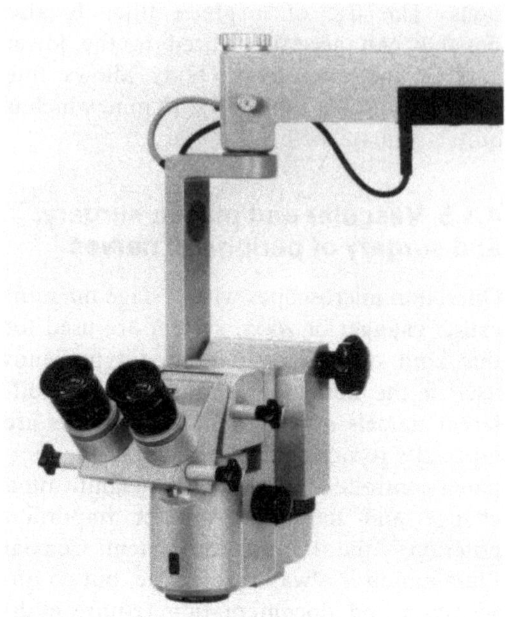

Fig. 99. Short zoom operation microscope with tiltable tube, with illuminator carrier C and slit illuminator.

zoom system, and different illumination systems. The older types Opmi 6 and 6 H offer magnifications from $0.5\times$ to $2.5\times$. The new type (Fig. 99) is more compact and has a zooming range from $0.5\times$ to $2.0\times$. The motorized zoom system has a manual override. The latest models feature swing-in (green) filters. The illumination system of the operation microscope Opmi 6 S corresponds to that of the Opmi 6, while those of Opmi 6 F and 6 H are different. The operation microscope 6 F is equipped with a fiber optics system for illumination of the operating field, and Opmi 6 H with a 12 V 100 W halogen lamp, which makes it especially suitable for documentation.

c) Operation microscopes Opmi 7 D and 8 D. Double microscopes offer surgeon and assistant the same viewing direction on the operating field. The two types differ in an additional assistant's microscope of the Opmi 8 D, which can be mounted on either side of the microscope (Fig. 100).

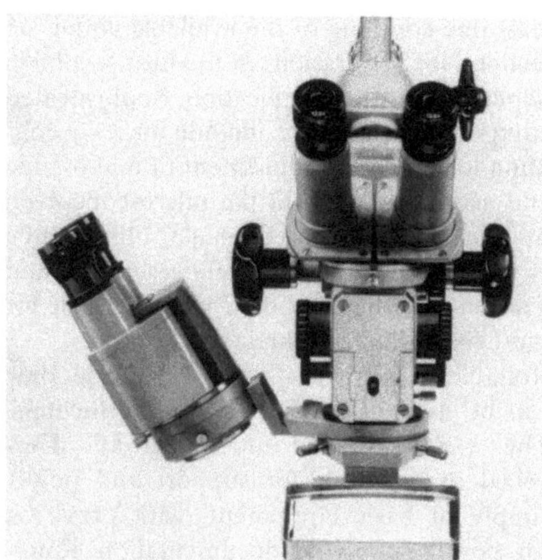

Fig. 98. Operation microscope Opmi 1 with assistant's microscope (27° inclination) and operating field magnifier.

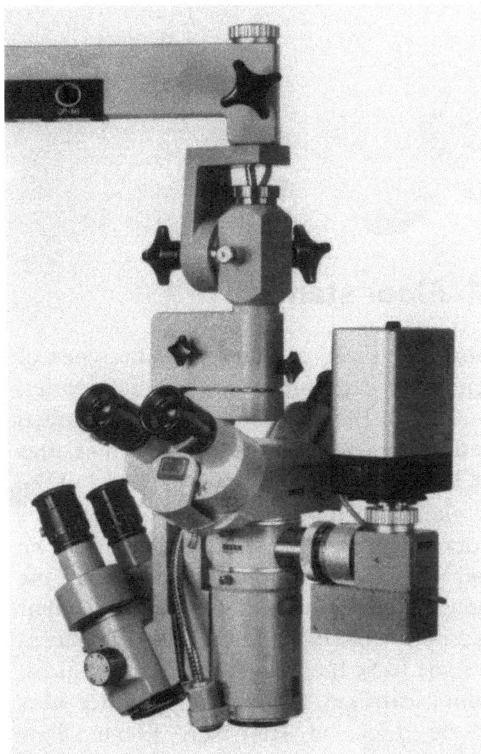

Fig. 100. Double microscope Opmi 8 D with assistant's microscope.

4.2 Frequently used couplings

Frequently used couplings and the $x-y$ coupling are listed in the following table.

Table 10. Survey of couplings

Type	Inclination [°]	Length [mm]
K 0/120	0	120
0/235	0	235
K 0/parallel	60	162
90/60	90	60
90/260	90	260
120/76 without gear control	120	76
120/76 with gear control	120	76

Fig. 101 shows some of the couplings listed in Table 10, Fig. 102 the $x-y$ coupling. Except for ENT and cerebral surgery it is required for sophisticated equipment in all disciplines. This coupling allows ± 25 mm shift of the microscope with accessories in two mutually perpendicular directions; it is automatically set to central position for rapid alignment of the instrument before surgical treatment at a speed of 5 mm/s. For reasons of stability the $x-y$ coupling can only be used on motorized stands or ceiling mounts.

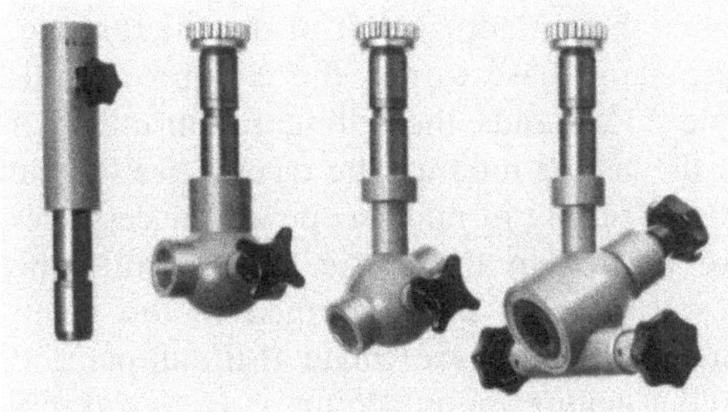

Fig. 101. Couplings

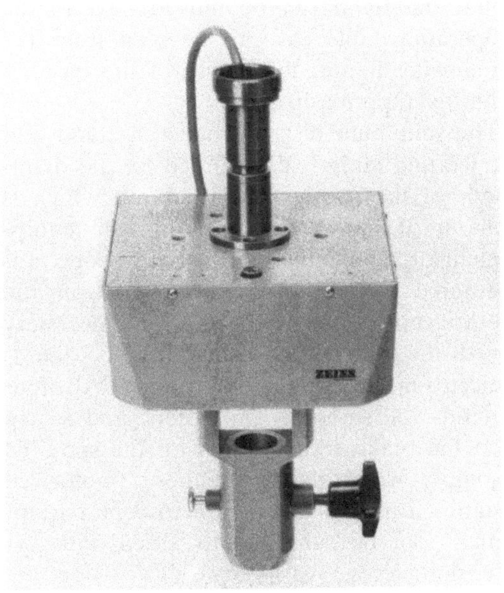

Fig. 102. $x-y$ coupling for motorized stands or ceiling mounts with automatic setting to central position.

5 Stands

Operation microscopes with components and accessories are mounted on stands by means of couplings, connecting pieces (see preceding chapter) and two or three carrier arms fitted to the carriage which slides up and down the stand's column and is used for coarse height adjustment of the microscope. The stand base carries the column of rollable floor stands, the ceiling mount unit that of the ceiling mount. The receptacles for the power supply of microscope and accessories are located in the carrier arms, while the power supplies are contained in the stand base or in the anchor plate at the upper end of the ceiling mount column. Heavy transformers add to the stability of the rollable floor stands. The stand base is so designed that the stand can be moved next to the operating table. As can be seen from the following figures the height of the bases is limited (approx. 50 cm).

The minimum distance between stand and operating table is determined by the diameter of the slender stand column which is about 55 mm. When installing the equipment or supplementing the microscope, additional weights can be provided in the outriggers for balancing. This is not necessary with the (older) electro-hydraulic or (latest) electro-mechanical ceiling mounts. All floor stands roll smoothly on casters, and a step on the brake secures them on the spot. To comply with safety regulations, motorized stands carrying heavy microscope equipment can be subsequently fitted with extension pieces.

5.1 Floor stands

Floor stands are available for all types of microscope equipment with accessories. There are 1.88 m stands and motorized stands. The column of the first measures 1.88 m from the floor to the upper end of the column, and can be rolled through the doors of operating theaters without having to be tilted. All 1.88 m floor stands have the following basic features in common: their design principle is the same, and they accept the same basic modules such as carrier arms, column, carriage, and base. The differences will be discussed later. All 1.88 m floor stands are equipped with a vertically adjustable, lockable safety ring on the column which must be secured before starting surgical treatment, so that the deepest point of the operation microscope does not come into contact with patient or operating field. All "Standard" and "Universal" stands are available for different mains voltages (100 to 240 V) and frequencies (50 or 60 Hz).

The motorized stands are of entirely different design. Their stability is higher, they are more compact, made to carry heavier equipment. As microsurgical equipment is becoming more sophisticated, the extra-heavy motorized floor stands are gaining more and more popularity, of course, besides the ceiling mounts. The vertical travel of motorized floor stands and ceiling mounts is motorized.

5.1.1 1.88 m stands

a) Standard I. A simple stand, used especially in ophthalmology, with electrical power supply only for coaxial illumination, homogeneous and slit illuminator (Fig. 103). If a fiber optics system is used, as, for instance, prescribed in the USA, the complete electrical assembly is removed and replaced by a cover plate on the front surface of the stand base. The supply voltages can be used singly or in combination at rated 6 or 8.5 V overload.

b) Standard II. It has different electrical equipment from the Standard I. It contains a power supply for an electronic flash (160 Ws), and a 24 V power supply for a motor drive which can also be subsequently fitted (Fig. 104). Hand- or foot-panel-controlled, this motor drive at the head of the stand [7 a] silently moves the microscope carrier arm up and down at a speed of 5 mm/s.

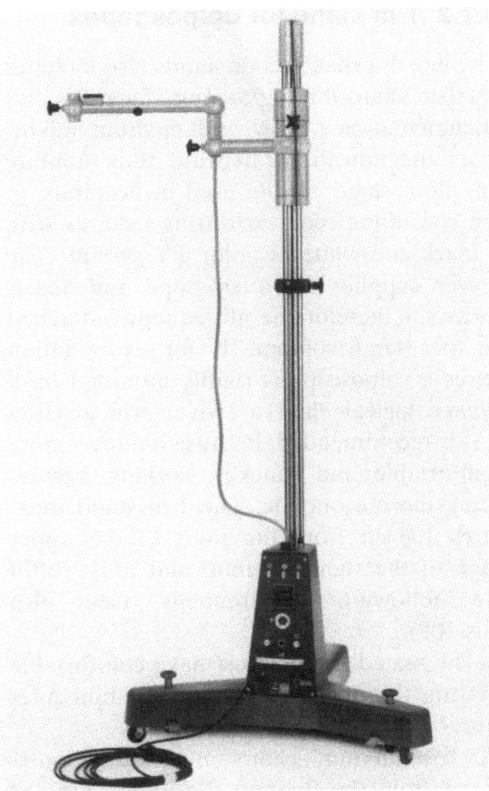

Fig. 104. Standard II stand with attachable motor drive.

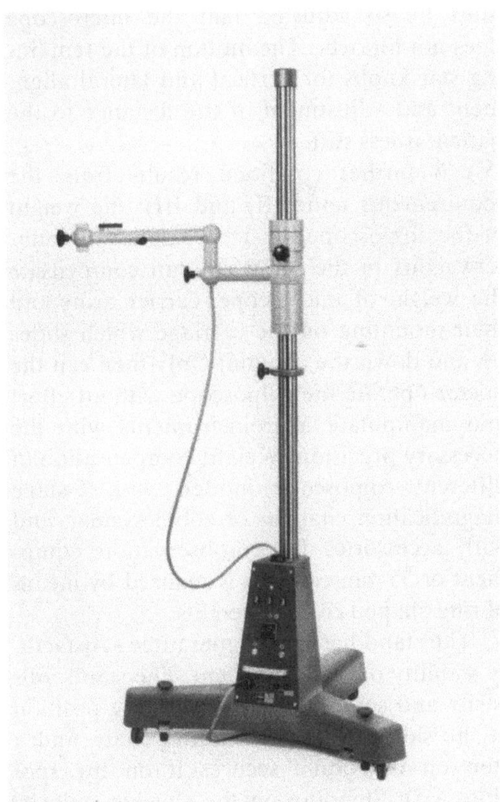

Fig. 103. Front view of the Standard I stand.

c) Universal. In the stand's base individual push-button overload switches are provided for each of the three compatible illuminators. Which power line is supplied with overvoltage is indicated by the overload key which lights up. A higher power input to the stand base is necessary, but this fact is irrelevant to the user. The other outputs of the stand base correspond to those of the Standard II. The "Universal" stand accepts the three conventional illuminators, an optional electronic flash (160 Ws), the motor drive of the microscope column, and the supply for motorized focusing and zoom actions of the microscope. A remote footswitch control permits overloading of operative illuminators.

5.1.2 1-m stand for colposcopes

The line of rollable floor stands also includes the 1-m stand for colposcopic diagnosis and documentation at low and medium microscope magnifications. Because of its mobility this floor stand can be used in hospitals, in the consulting room or during lectures with a black-and-white or color TV system. The power supplies for microscope and accessories can therefore be subsequently attached to the stand column. If for examination series a colposcope is rigidly mounted on a gynaecological chair a swivel arm (section 5.5) is recommended, because it allows more comfortable and quicker working besides being more economic. The 1-m stand measures 106 cm from the floor to the upper edge of the stand column, and must fulfill the following requirements (see also Fig. 105):

I) The seated doctor must have comfortable viewing through the colposcope's binocular tube.

II) Examination chairs measure approx. 85 cm from the floor to the upper edge of the top surface. The height of the top sur-

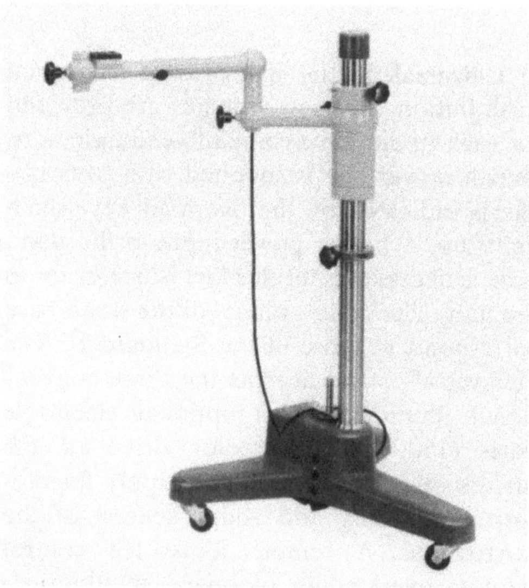

Fig. 105. Rollable 1-m stand for colposcopes.

face of older models is not variable. The patient's position with regard to the colposcope can be adjusted within certain limits. It is faster and more precise if the doctor adjusts the microscope laterally, vertically, its viewing direction and axial focusing. This also applies to more comfortable examination chairs with motorized vertical adjustment.

III) A colposcope must be mobile and therefore have lightweight moving parts (microscope itself, accessories, and carrier arms). Stability, durability, and operating safety set the lower weight limit. The microscope must move smoothly in its mounting and in the points of rotation of the carrier arms. The rotary and swivel motions can be individually adjusted for the most convenient working position with the star knobs. The friction of the microscope's horizontal axis of rotation must be so adjusted that the microscope does not tilt over. The motion of the remaining star knobs for vertical and lateral alignment and adjustment of the distance to the patient is less stiff.

IV) A further condition results from the requirements under II) and III): the weight of the colposcope must be balanced. Counterweights in the stand column compensate the weight of microscope, carrier arms and their mounting on the carriage which slides up and down the column. Only then can the doctor operate the colposcope without effort and manipulate microinstruments with the necessary precision. Weight compensation of different colposcope models with 5-stage magnification changer or zoom system, and with accessories for co-observation equipment or 35 mm cameras is realized by means of ring-shaped counterweights.

V) The stand base must guarantee satisfactory stability of the instrument. The stand rolls easily and smoothly to the working position at the side of the examination chair, and a step on the brake secures it on the spot (Fig. 105). Stepping on the shackle unlocks the brake. The heavy stand base with the

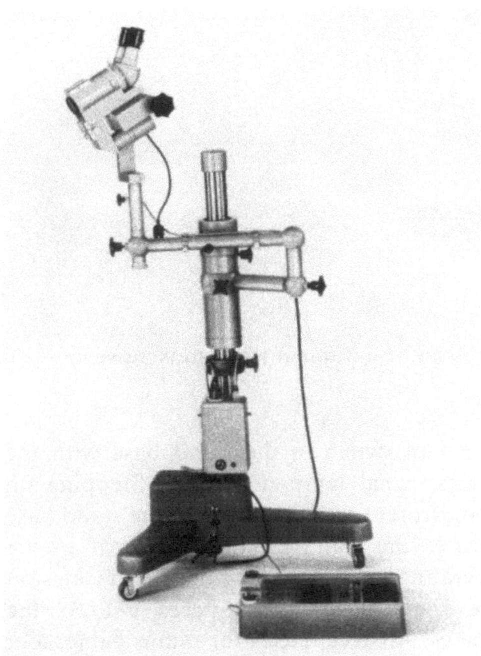

Fig. 106. 1-m stand with electrical power supply for colposcope 6 and foot-panel control.

electrical power supply of the microscope's illumination system and the heavy column guarantee vibration-free stability of the microscope, even with extensive accessories and at high magnifications.

VI) The Opmi 1 colposcope is equipped with a 5-stage magnification changer. The zoom colposcope (Opmi 6, Fig. 106) needs an additional power supply for the microscope's zoom and axial focusing motors. Both motors can be controlled from a foot panel, which frees the surgeon's hands for manipulations of the microinstruments. The power supply unit is mounted on the stand column beneath the ring limiting the vertical movement of the carriage.

VII) The stand base accepts different electrical assemblies. Via dovetails an electronic flash can be fitted to the microscope bottom for the documentation of findings. A stand base with an 80 Ws power supply unit is available for the electronic flash.

5.1.3 Motor stands

When it is desirable to attach extensive and heavy microscope equipment and accessories, and when a ceiling mount must be excluded because mounting is needed in different operating theater the use of motor stands is recommended. Such extensive equipment as must be mounted either on the ceiling mount or on a motor stand is required, for instance, in ophthalmic microsurgery of retina and vitreous body, or in hand surgery where the microscope is usually a triploscope which increases the weight of the equipment to such an extent that lighter and less sturdy stands cannot be used. Apart from different power supplies (100 to 120 W, 60 Hz or 200 to 240 V, 50 Hz) there are two basic types of motor stands: 1) stands with mechanical drive for coarse height adjustment and positioning of the microscope, and 2) stands which are adjusted to working position once and for all by suitable intermediate pieces when installed. The vertical motorized travel of both stands for precision adjustment is covered at 15 mm/s.

Only with the microscope Opmi 7 and 8 is the vertical adjustment with the stand at the same time the focusing motion. These two microscopes are primarily used in ophthalmic microsurgery of the anterior segments of the eye, and additional focusing facilities are not necessary. Microscopes with 5-stage magnification changer (Opmi 1) and zoom system (Opmi 6) are most frequently mounted on motor stands. Both instruments allow the surgeon to focus the microscope axially: manually with a control on one side of Opmi 1, and motorized on the Opmi 6. Axial focusing is necessary whenever the microscope is tilted around its horizontal axis; the vertical adjustment of the stand can then not be used also to adjust the microscope to deep operating fields.

Both motor stands have the same 400 VA/ 80 Ws electrical assembly to power the

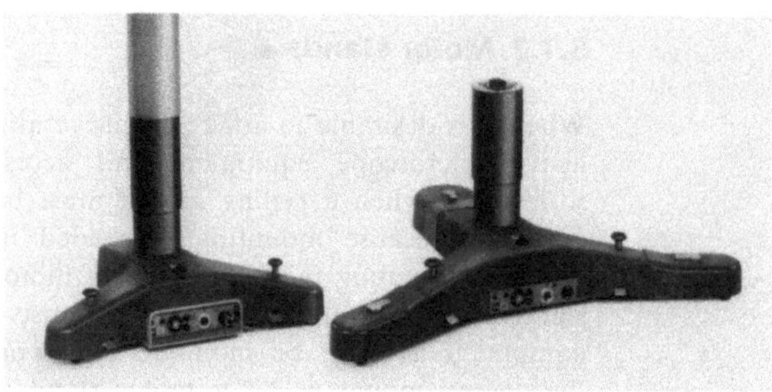

Fig. 107. Motor stand base. Standard version (left), and stand base with outriggers to increase the stability of the microscope with heavy accessories.

microscope's illumination system, cameras for still or cine photography, and the motors of zoom system and precision focusing of zoom microscopes, as well as the motorized ±30° slit lamp for ophthalmology. All these functions can be controlled from a hand or foot panel. The on-off switch of both models is a foot switch in the stand base with the mains signal lamp next to it. Stepping on two further switches on top of the stand base secures the stand on the spot next to the operating table. Stepping on the shackles on the front of the stand bases unlocks the brakes. All receptacles for mains cable, foot or hand switch and electronic flash (Fig. 107) are arranged on the front surface of the stand base, and so are the electrical fuses.

Two or sometimes three carrier arms are part of the stand. The carrier arm on the stand column carries at the bottom two potentiometers for lamp voltage adjustment of two separate microscope lamps for illumination of the operating field. Pressing down the pushbuttons between the knobs switches the lamps to overload; the keys light.

With the star knobs at the side of the carrier arms these are secured or loosened for rotation about the vertical axis. With these knobs different amounts of friction can be adjusted between the two limiting positions, for instance, for turning the microscope on the carrier arm in the adjusted position without danger of disadjustment when the instrument is inadvertently touched.

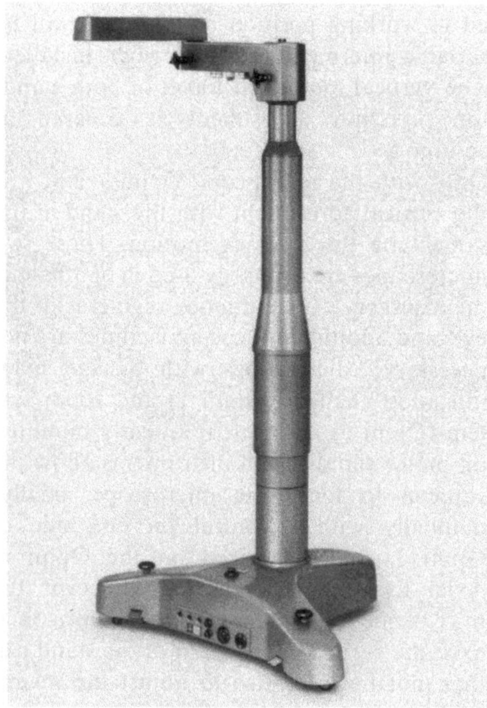

Fig. 108. Motor stand without continuous mechanical height adjustment.

a) Motor stand without continuous mechanical height adjustment (Fig. 108). 300 mm extension is possible by means of an intermediate piece. The motorized travel covers a range of 150 mm at a speed of 5 mm/s.

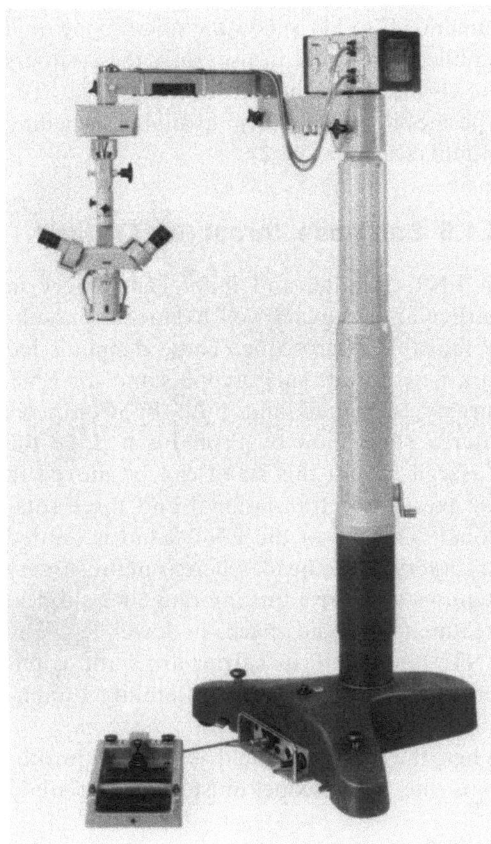

Fig. 109. Motor stand with crank for continuous height adjustment of the stand column.

b) Motor stand with mechanical height adjustment. The height of this stand (Fig. 109) is coarsely adjusted by a crank at the side of the stand column. The vertical adjusting range is 390 mm. Additional motorized travel within a range of 150 mm at a speed of 5 mm/s is possible.

5.1.4 Mobile floor stand for neurosurgery

A special development for neurosurgery made by Contraves of Zurich upon the suggestion of Prof. Yaşargil, offering extraordinary versatility of microscope adjustment. The surgical technique Yaşargil developed, for instance, for intercranial surgery of an aneurysm requires high microscope magnification. This in turn means limited depth of focus of the microscope. The soft tissue yields to microinstruments and moves out of focus; the microscope must be re-focused. Putting down one or both instruments for manual re-focusing of the microscope would be too time-consuming. Yaşargil therefore suggested an adjustable mouth switch which when on disengages electromagnetic clutches in the microscope mount and allows the surgeon to adjust the microscope to the desired position with his teeth.

Besides extraordinary mobility all microscope adjustments must be *smooth*. For this purpose the microscope's weight must be well balanced by counterweights for transverse and vertical adjustment, tilt, and rotation. When the microscope is equipped with co-observation and documentation instruments which vary depending on application and requirements, a sophisticated system of tares is necessary. One specific piece of microscope equipment is tared once. The more careful the balancing is done, the more easily can the microscope be moved in all axes. More effort is needed if the adjustment is not correct. The use of sterilization cloths may make minor corrections to adjustments necessary, but after some training these can be carried out by a member of the staff in the operating theater.

Although neurosurgical procedures require a high degree of maneuverability, the microscope must also be lockable in every position set. This is achieved by magnetic clutches in the cylinders on the stand joints, which can be operated by means of two different switching systems. With the switch in one of the two handles all possible settings in the six axes can be unlocked and locked, while the mouth switch can only be used for the three translational adjustments. Fig. 110 shows a microscope Opmi 1 on the stand coupling and the ranges of maneuverability.

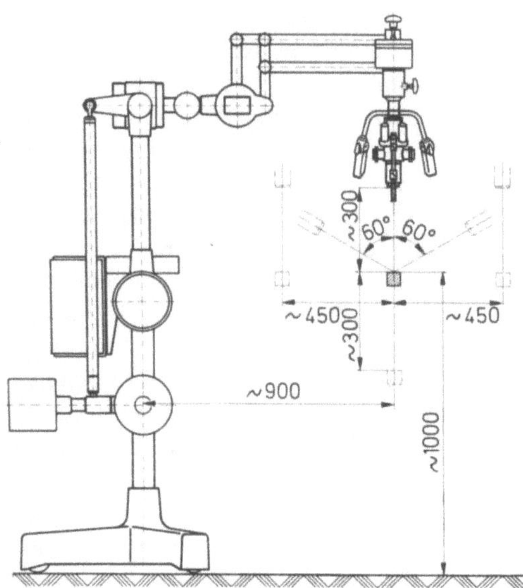

Fig. 110. Adjusting and tilting range of the mobile stand for neurosurgery.

The power supply unit feeds the microscope lamp, the microscope motors for precision focusing and magnification changer (Opmi 6), and the "Urban" and "Beaulieu" cine cameras. Fig. 111 shows the microscope on a mobile floor stand in use; only the contours are visible under the sterile cloths.

The mobile stand is also available as ceiling mount (see para. 5.2.2).

5.1.5 Ear, nose, throat (ENT) stand

In ENT, middle, and inner ear surgery in particular requires a well balanced, smoothly movable microscope. These demands led to a new mobile microscope stand for ENT surgery, designed and built by Contraves after a suggestion by Prof. Fisch. Like the Yaşargil mount this stand can be moved in six axes, three translational and three rotational. The use of the ENT stand is limited to surgery of the head, whereas neurosurgery requires a larger adjusting range for surgical treatment of head, back, or lower leg. The ENT stand itself, its carrier arms and counterweights are therefore differently dimensioned.

When the operating field is focused in otology, the microscope must often be tilted

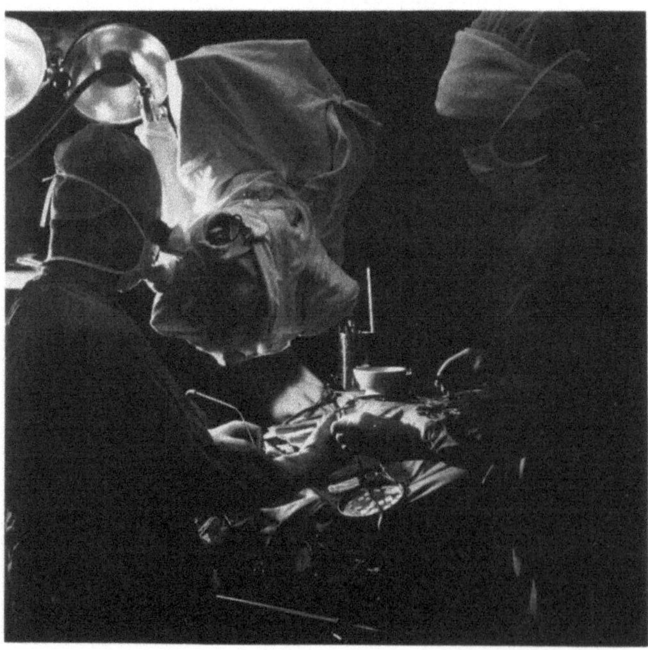

Fig. 111. Mobile stand for neurosurgery in use. (Photograph by courtesy of Messrs. Aesculap)

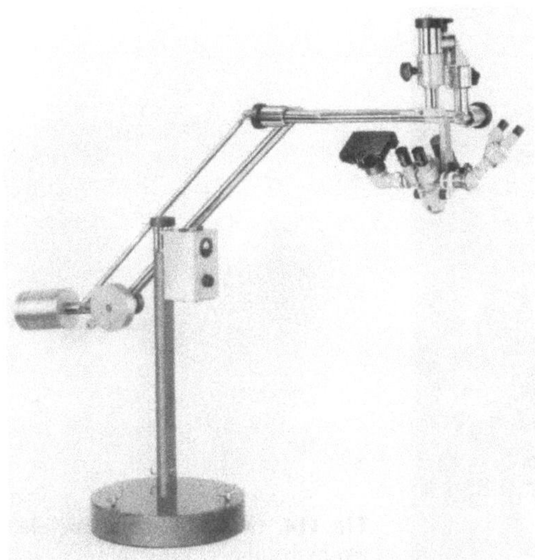

Fig. 112. Mobile stand for ENT surgery after Fisch.

5.2 Ceiling mounts

As microsurgery progressed, space around the operating table became more and more crowded by instrumentation and personnel, which in the end even interfered with the work of surgeon and assistant. The three major elements around the table are the stand with the operating microscope, the equipment for anaesthesia, and the instrument table. Ceiling mounts are gaining more and more popularity because they help unclutter the floor space of the operating room and can accommodate heavy accessories which are the rule, for instance, for vitreous surgery. Ceiling mounts have the further advantage that the microscope is readily brought into working position above the operating table. They have the disadvantage of being stationary so that they cannot be used in different operating theaters. The ceiling height must be between 2.9 and 4.2 m, a requirement which is certainly always fulfilled. Furthermore, a normal load of 4000 N and a moment of 5000 Nm must be considered, which are fed into the ceiling, and the architect must provide an anchor plate in the load-bearing ceiling.

quickly and easily in all directions, without any danger of "tiltover" which would require repositioning.

These demands led to the development of the ENT stand after Prof. Fisch shown in Fig. 112. The stand accepts, of course, accessories for co-observation and documentation. Fig. 113 shows the stand in clinical use.

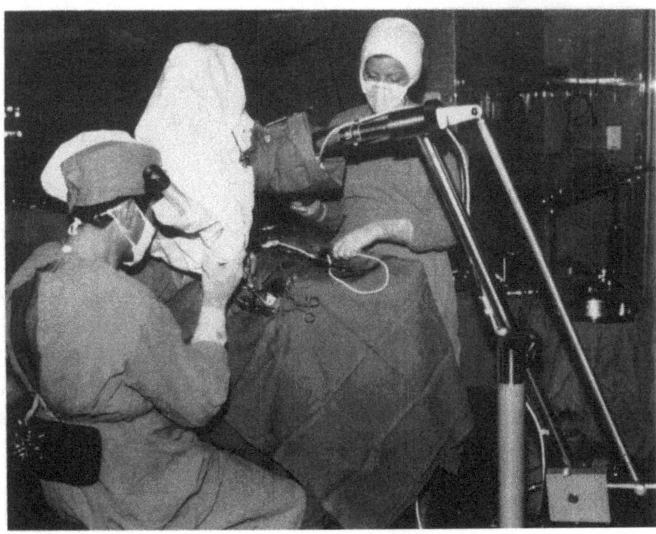

Fig. 113. ENT stand in use.

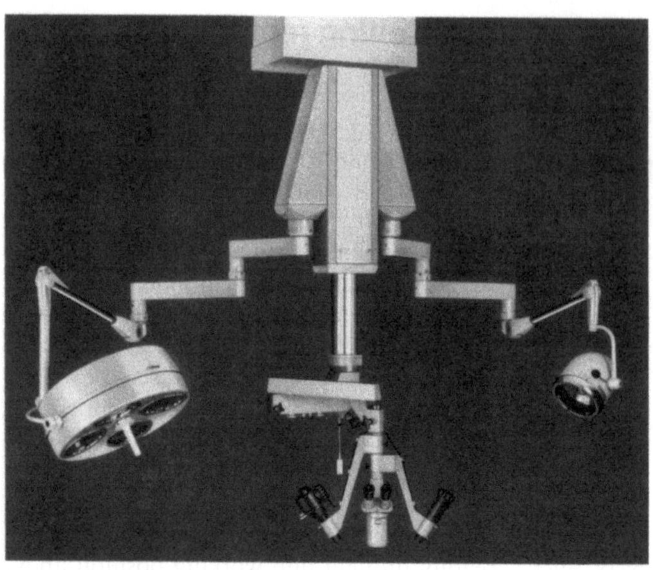

Fig. 114. Overall view of the electro-hydraulic ceiling mount with operating lamps.

5.2.1 Electro-hydraulic and electro-mechanical ceiling mounts

The first ceiling mount developed by Zeiss was electro-hydraulic (Fig. 114), so named because the microscope is pneumatically lifted and lowered. Further development led to the electro-mechanical ceiling mount

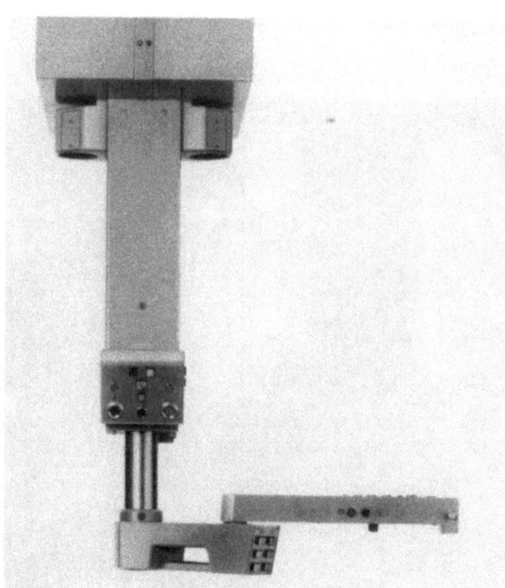

Fig. 115. New electro-mechanical ceiling mount.

which has all the proven functions of the former model and some new ones (Fig. 115). The 500 mm vertical-focusing adjustment is motorized at a speed of 3 mm/s or, optionally, 4 mm/s, or manual. In the latter case the microscope equipment is, of course, well balanced by adjustable weights for smooth maneuverability. To protect the patient the adjustment is continuous and lockable. The power supply facilities for accessories have been expanded. Besides 6 V and 12 V AC for the microscope lamps, 12 V DC are now available for motorized focusing and magnification change. 12 V DC are also available for the motorized operation slit lamp, and 7.2 V and 3.6 V DC for the "Beaulieu" cine camera with automatic diaphragm control. In addition there are 12 V DC for the 35 mm camera with motorized film transport, 24 V AC, e.g. for thermo-coagulator, and 7 V AC for an ophthalmoscope. The connection of a microphone is possible, and different functions (e.g. camera release) can be foot- or hand-panel-controlled, either alternatively or simultaneously. An electronic flash is compatible, and a mains socket can be provided. The control panel can be mounted on the lower part of the stand

(Fig. 115) or externally on the wall of the operating theater.

The following provisions are necessary before a ceiling mount can be mounted: an anchor plate or, in case of high ceilings, an intermediate plate in the load-bearing ceiling to anchor the ceiling column. The center of the mounting plate should coincide with the center line of the operating table, and should be approximately 500 mm above the center of the head rest. Only then can the microscope with its two carrier arms be adjusted to the various operating fields, and the two laterally mounted operating lamps swung into optimum working position without interfering with the microscope.

Preparations on the part of the builder must also include the laying of a tube of at least 22 mm internal diameter for the power supply line to the column. Tubes for supply lines must also be provided for rollable operating chairs with control elements, a wall console, a microphone center, for motorized control of the operating table, and for operating lamps on the ceiling mount, that means a maximum of 5 tubes.

The height at which the ceiling mount is fitted depends on the height of the operating table, the most frequently used objective focal length, and the type of microscope equipment including the couplings. This also decides whether an intermediate plate is necessary for high ceilings.

A separate leaflet includes all details which must be considered for the fitting of a ceiling mount.

When planning a new operating room it is recommended to provide swivel-mounted operating lamps on opposite sides of the ceiling mount, for instance, the Hanaulux types "Hamburg", "Universal" or "London" (Fig. 114).

5.2.2 Mobile ceiling mount for neurosurgery

The mobile mount described in para. 5.1.4 can also be mounted on the ceiling (Fig. 116)

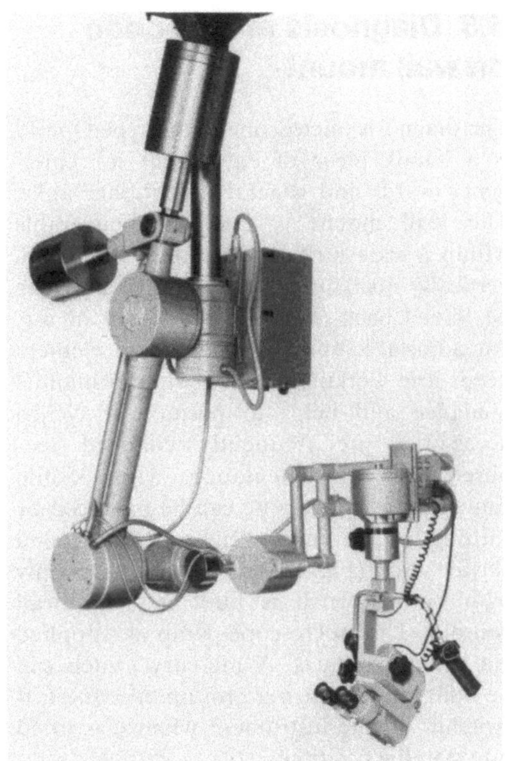

Fig. 116. Mobile ceiling mount for neurosurgery.

which unclutters the floor space around the operating table. But the counterweights for balancing microscope and accessories are not as easily accessible as on the floor stand. Furthermore, the ceiling mount is stationary and its use restricted to one operating theater. The functions described in para. 5.1.4 are the same for both types of mount.

The necessary preparations on the part of the builder include the anchor plate for the ceiling mount and the laying of the tubes for the electrical power lines.

5.2.3 Mobile ENT ceiling mount

The floor stand for otorhinolaryngology described in para. 5.1.5, is also available as ceiling mount. The statements concerning the mobile operation microscope stand for neurosurgery also apply to this mount.

5.3 Diagnosis microscope on wall mount

The diagnosis microscope of the type Opmi 9 is a handy piece of equipment for emergency wards and general practitioner alike. The wall mount is easily maneuverable within a wide range (horizontally 1350 mm, vertically 1000 mm; see Fig. 117), and can be folded back (Fig. 118) when not in use. An adjustable spring as balancing element keeps it in working position without manual guidance and helps to position it. When accessories are frequently changed (co-observation, documentation with 35 mm camera), the microscope can be balanced by shifting an additional weight on the second carrier arm (Fig. 118). The power supply with on-off switch is built into the wall console. The microscope lamp is supplied via sliding contacts. A mercury switch can be built into the carrier arm upon request; it switches off the instrument when it is lifted into standby position.

The operation microscope Opmi 9 on wall mount has exchangeable objectives, binocu-

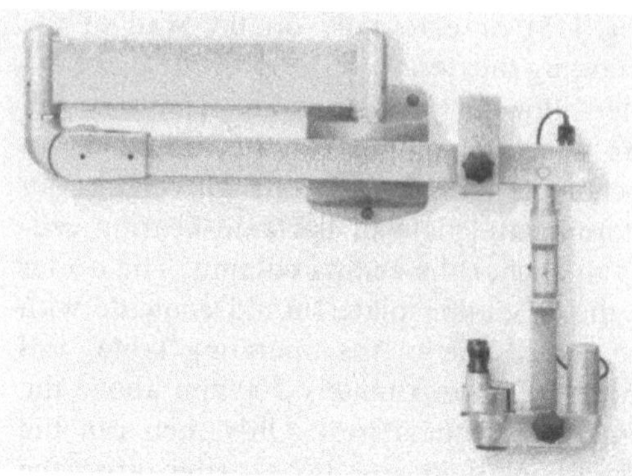

Fig. 118. Diagnosis microscope Opmi 9 on wall swivel arm in standby position.

lar tube, and eyepiece pairs, and an additional 3-stage magnification changer and objective focusing. It is not only a proven diagnosis microscope but also the best choice for post-operative examination and treatment of seated or recumbent patients, for minor surgery, and for training and instruction.

5.4 Diagnosis microscope for ENT diagnostic unit

The operation microscope Opmi 9 with accessories is also a simple, efficient, and economic microscope for ENT emergency wards and practitioners, for minor surgery and for post-operative control. It has all the essential features for the purpose, namely built-in coaxial illumination, easy objective and eyepiece exchange (which also changes the magnification), objective focusing, and 3-stage magnification change. The microscope can be mounted on a rollable floor stand (para. 5.1.1), the wall mount (section 5.3), or a special column integral with a diagnostic unit (Fig. 119). This permits the microscope to be used in accordance with biotechnical principles. The microscope is suspended from two carrier arms which can be easily and smoothly moved up and down

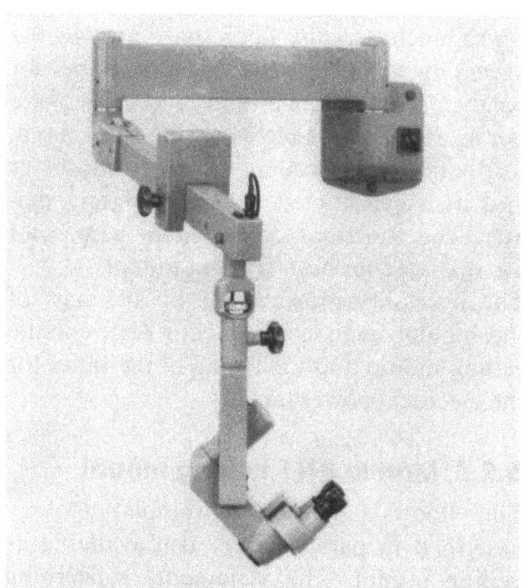

Fig. 117. Diagnosis microscope Opmi 9 on wall swivel arm in working position.

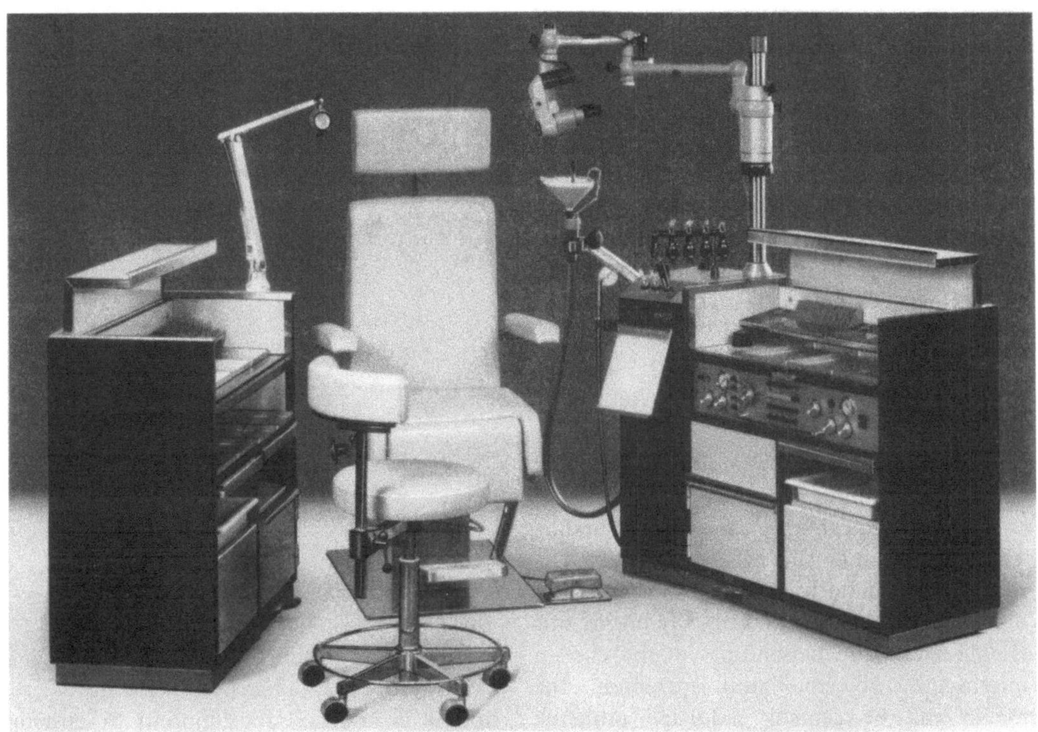

Fig. 119. Diagnosis microscope Opmi 9 part of an ENT diagnostic unit. (Courtesy of Messrs. Atmos, Lenzkirch)

the column on the stand carriage owing to built-in counterweights.

5.5 Colposcope swivel arm

Swivel arms for different gynaecological examination chairs (tubular or compact design) can also be subsequently fitted without modification of the chair. Only a metal upright with clamps is required for tubular steel chairs (Fig. 120), and for compact chairs a holder for the upright which is supplied and fitted to the chair by the manufacturer.

The microscope lamp is supplied with power by a transformer in the main body of the swivel arm, which also carries the mode selector to switch the lamp to overload. A bubble on top of the arm serves to level the swivel arm during assembly.

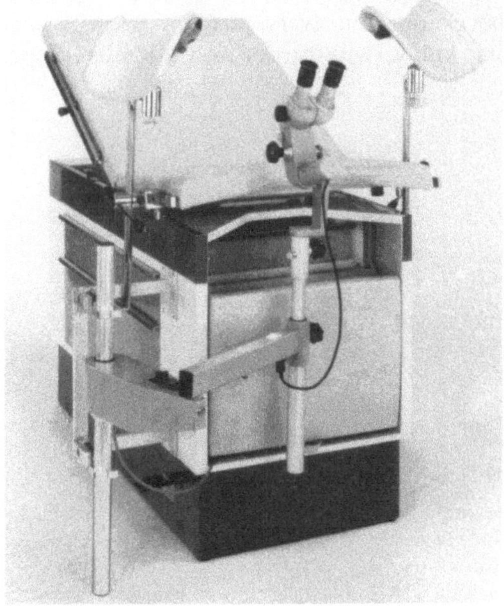

Fig. 120. Swivel arm for gynaecological examination chairs.

In standby position the swivel arm should hinder neither the patient nor the doctor. Easy and fast positioning for colposcopic examinations is ensured by the three vertical axes of rotation, the two carrier arms, and the telescope tube for vertical adjustment of the microscope (in addition to the adjusting capabilities of the swivel arm the microscope can be tilted around a horizontal axis and axially focused).

5.6 Table stand

The microscope can be mounted on table stands, for training purposes, for dissection, or for the inspection of microinstruments. The table stand (Fig. 121) consists of a rugged base plate for the column with pivoted microscope carrier arm. Owing to this simple setup and depending on the chosen microscope objective and specimen, the height can be coarsely adjusted and the microscope turned around the vertical axis of the pivot and the horizontal axis of the microscope carrier arm. The microscope can be clamped in every position set with the star knobs (with carrier arm the microscope

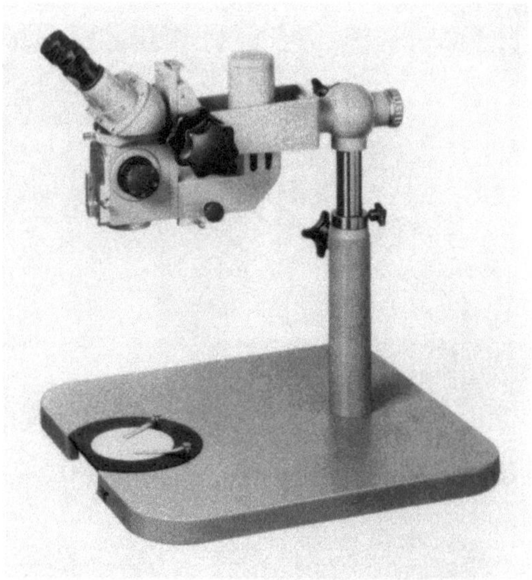

Fig. 121. Table stand with microscope Opmi 1.

can be tilted around a horizontal axis and axially focused; objective focusing is required in addition for Opmi 9). A circular recess in the base plate accepts mechanical or gliding stages. Specimen slides can, for instance, be fixed with attachable stage clips. Circular and rectangular base plates are available for the table stands.

6 Supplements and accessories

Accessories for operation microscopes include primarily assistant's microscopes, but in a wider sense also equipment for co-observation through the optics of the operation microscope, and, lastly, an ample selection of documentation systems. With the rapid expansion of microsurgery, documentation in particular is gaining more and more popularity and will be discussed in detail in chapter 8. Assistant's microscopes and co-observation devices are described below.

6.1 Beam splitters

It is one of the major advantages of the modular operation microscope system that new models as well as those which were supplied years ago and have been in use ever since can be subsequently fitted with a beam splitter between microscope body and binocular tube.

6.1.1 Beam splitter

The optical principle of the beam splitter is shown in Fig. 122: a cube in each of the microscope's two observation beam paths splits the light into two parts: one part is relayed upwards to the binocular tube but retains its entrance direction, the other one

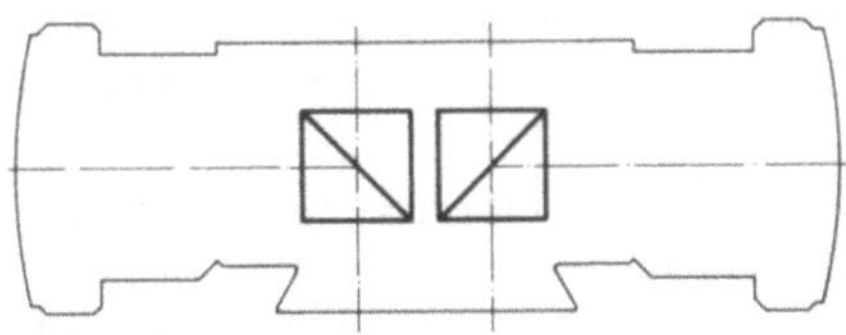

Fig. 122. Beam splitter (cross-sectional view).

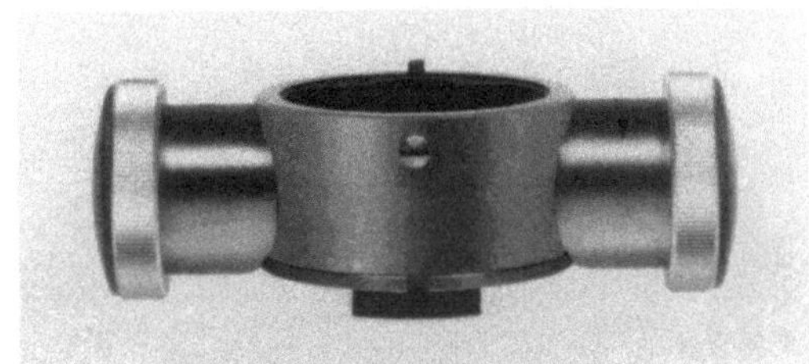

Fig. 123. Beam splitter 50.

is 90° laterally reflected. The beam splitter is shown in Fig. 123. It is available in two versions: a type 50 which reflects 50% of the light into each of the above-mentioned directions (losses due to reflection and absorption in the two cubes are negligible), and a type 70, especially for documentation, in that 70% of the two incident light beams are laterally reflected for use by documentation equipment. As the losses due to reflection and absorption are negligible, the remaining 30% are available for observation of the operating field.

As shown in Fig. 123 the mechanical design of the beam splitter's top surface corresponds to that of the microscope body to accommodate the binocular tube. Adapters for photography, cine, and TV systems or co-observation tubes can be attached the two ports on the side of the beam splitter. All attachments are secured by a knurled compression nut.

6.1.2 Stereo beam splitter

The above-mentioned beam splitter reflects the two observation beam paths laterally so that, for instance, a 35 mm camera can be used on one side, and a co-observation tube on the other. The stereo beam splitter serves another purpose. It offers at the same time to surgeon and assistant exactly the same direction of viewing on the operating field in that a large splitting cube is arranged above both beam paths which relays equal (energetically split) beam paths to both exists. Surgeon and assistant have thus the same

6.2 Assistant's microscope

With an assistant's microscope [10] the operating field seen by the surgeon and at the same time a somewhat larger field must be surveyed stereoscopically. The magnification available to the assistant is therefore lower. He can change the magnification with a 3-

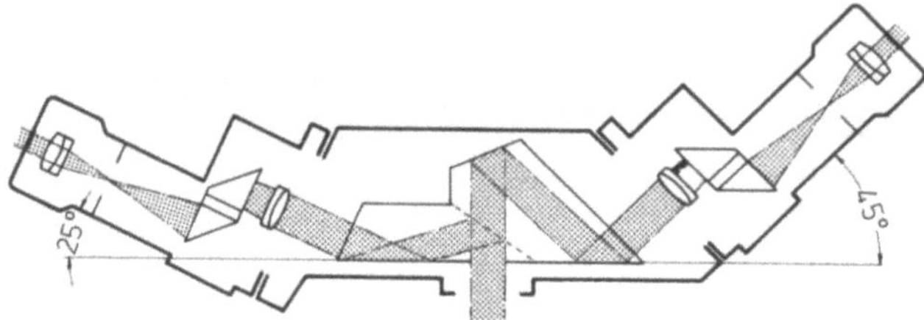

Fig. 124. Beam path of the stereo beam splitter.

stereo basis, and get the same stereoscopic impression of the object. Fig. 124 shows the optical principle of the system. A noticeable feature is the different angles at which the two exit surfaces of the prism cubes are tilted, but it is this design which guarantees the most favorable viewing angle for surgeon and assistant if different binocular tubes (straight or inclined) are used on the tilted microscope.

While the beam splitter can be used on all operation microscopes, the stereo beam splitter fits only onto the microscope types Opmi 2 and Opmi 7. The stereo beam splitter must cover both beam paths, a condition which is not fulfilled by all other microscopes because of the microscope holder. An older model of a zoom microscope Opmi 2 with stereo beam splitter is shown in Fig. 83.

The main fields of application of the stereo beam splitter are hand surgery, reconstructive surgery and neurosurgery, but it is finding more and more acceptance also in ophthalmology, for surgery of the anterior segments of the eye. Owing to its great advantages the stereo beam splitter has become an indispensable piece of equipment for training purposes.

stage Galilean magnification changer between microscope body and binocular tube (see para. 2.4.1), which can be subsequently fitted. The same accessories used on the main microscope, objectives, binocular tube, and eyepieces, also fit onto the assistant's microscope. The assistant's microscopes described below differ from the main microscopes only in the type of mounting and the angles their axes form with the main microscope.

6.2.1 Assistant's microscope on double microscopes

The double microscopes Opmi 5 and Opmi 8 for ophthalmic microsurgery feature assistant's microscopes which are separated from the main microscope but turned around the main microscope's vertical axis; both operation microscope types are used for surgery of the anterior segments of the eye. The axes of the assistant's microscopes form an angle of 27° with the axis of the main microscope. Fig. 125 shows the Opmi 5 double microscope after Harms.

An assistant's microscope has the great advantage that it can be turned within a wide range around the same axis as the main microscope, although its use is restricted to the anterior segments of the eye because of the large angle between assistant's and main microscope.

Like the main microscope the assistant's microscope of Opmi 5 has a 5-stage magnification changer. The assistant's microscopes

be arranged as near to the main microscope as possible. The following types of assistant's microscopes have evolved, which also fulfill further requirements:

a) Assistant's microscope 27°. This microscope [7 b] is of excellent maneuverability due to the wide turning capacity around the main microscope, and additional turning

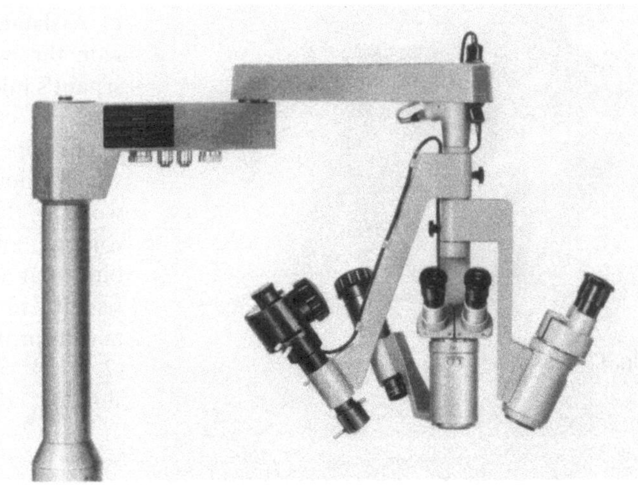

Fig. 125. Assistant's microscope of new model Opmi 8 operation microscope after Harms with homogeneous and slit illuminator.

for the first double zoom microscope systems also had zoom systems, but this design principle was soon abandoned because the assistant does not need the same (large) zooming range as the surgeon. Owing to the large angle between assistant's microscope and axis of the main microscope the focal plane seen by the assistant does not coincide with that seen by the surgeon. However, since the equipment described here is exclusively intended for surgery of the anterior segments of the eye, this is not disturbing.

6.2.2 Assistant's microscopes on the main microscope

For microsurgery other than ophthalmic the angle between assistant's and main microscope's axes should be as small as possible, which means the assistant's microscope must

capacity of the binocular tube about the microscope axis. It can be subsequently fitted to the main microscope with a carrier ring and a holder (Fig. 126) on one side of the main microscope, and easily set to the assistant's optimum working position. The angle between the two microscopes is, however, quite large, between 30° and 27°, depending on the focal length of the main microscope objective (150 to 200 mm). This disadvantage is acceptable as long as the operating field is flat. This type of assistant's microscope is neither intended nor suited for surgery in narrow body cavities, but can be fitted any time to an existing main microscope.

b) Assistant's microscope 16°. This microscope is mounted at the side of the main microscope body at an angle of 90° to the surgeon's viewing direction. Compared with

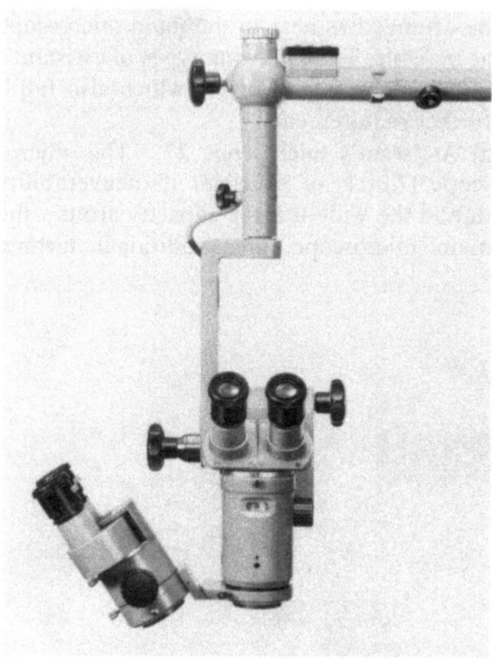

Fig. 126. Assistant's microscope 27°.

the 27° assistant's microscope, this results in a smaller viewing angle between 20 and 16°, depending on the focal length of the main microscope objective (150 to 200 mm). Once set the position of the microscope is unchangeable.

One assistant's microscope can be mounted on either side of the main microscope forming a triploscope for special applications (Fig. 127).

c) Assistant's microscope 8°. Compared with the two afore-mentioned types this assistant's microscope has the following advantages: it can be subsequently fitted to the microscope body by means of a double ring, which allows the assistant to turn it to the working direction he wants. In addition to rotation around the main microscope, the binocular tube can be turned about the assistant's microscope axis. It offers the assistant approximately the same viewing angle (7 to 9°) on the operating field as the surgeon, depending on the main micro-

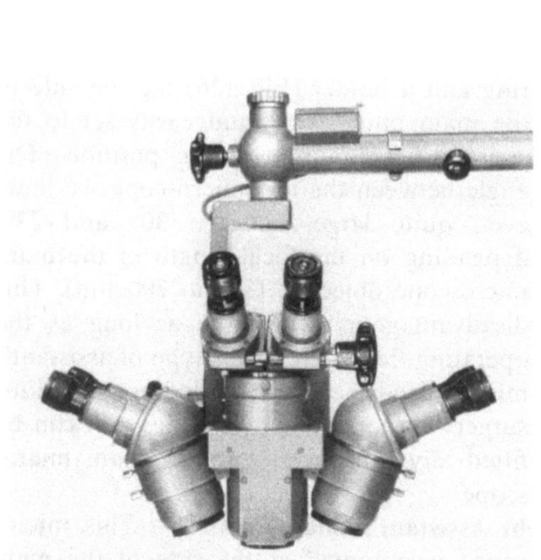

Fig. 127. An assistant's microscope 19° on each side of the main microscope.

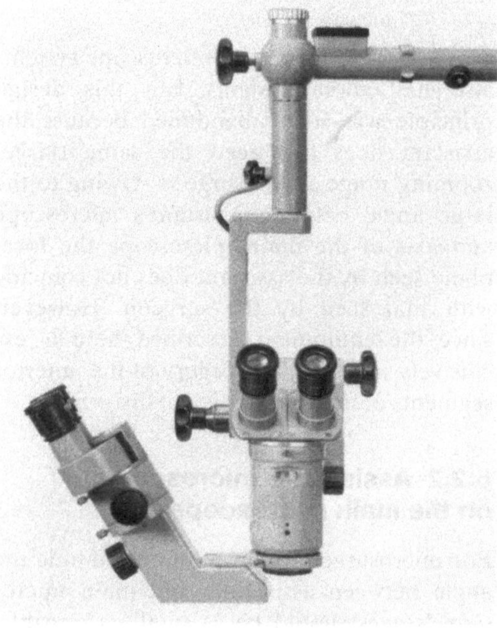

Fig. 128. Assistant's microscope 8°.

scope's objective focal length. Fig. 128 shows this assistant's microscope.

Last but not least this microscope has a built-in ± 6.5 mm focusing device.

As mentioned before, all three assistant's microscopes can be equipped with 3-stage magnification changers.

6.3 Co-observation equipment

Co-observation equipment [8 a] differs essentially from the above-mentioned assistant's microscopes. The latter have the same stereo basis as the main microscopes, i.e. they offer assistant and surgeon basically the same stereoscopic impression of the operating field. This is not true of co-observation equipment with one exception, but even therefore stereo basis and stereoscopic impression are limited. Co-observation equipment is always mounted via a beam splitter. Surgeon and assistant must accept the unavoidable light losses, but have the great advantage that the axes of co-observation device and main microscope coincide so that surgeon and assistant see the operating field at exactly the same angle.

Within a certain range all co-observation systems can be turned to a specific position, which changes the position of the image as well. To offer the co-observer a correct survey of and orientation capability to the operating field, all systems are provided with a device to rotate the image of the operating field so that it corresponds to the co-observer's viewing direction without co-observation system.

All co-observation devices can be attached to one of the ports of the beam splitter. Another co-observation system or an adapter for documentation equipment can be accommodated on the opposite port. Co-observation equipment is therefore used not only for visitors, but also for training and instruction in operation techniques and, with certain restrictions, even for assistance of the instrument nurse or the assistant surgeon.

6.3.1 Monocular co-observation systems

The image seen through monocular co-observation systems is *not* stereoscopic, but this is not absolutely necessary for co-observation.

a) Short co-observation tube. The optical principle is shown in Fig. 129. The "parallel"

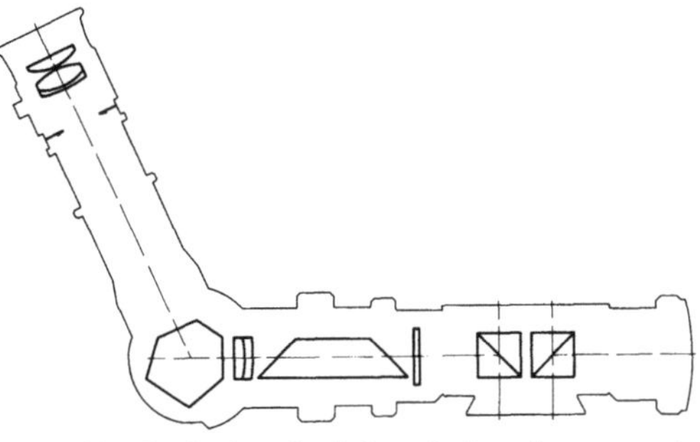

Fig. 129. Optical principle of the short co-observation tube.

light beams from the beam splitter fall on a dove prism for image rotation. This prism can be rotated through 360° (180° would be quite sufficient, but image rotation without mechanical stop is preferable for practical work).

Behind the image rotation prism a tube objective is arranged, as well as a prism which reflects the primary beam twice through 65°, and brings the image to a more comfortable observation position. The tube objective produces an intermediate image which can be observed re-enlarged by means of an eyepiece. The tube objective has a focal length of 160 mm. With a 160 mm binocular tube and the same eyepieces, e.g. 12.5×, co-observer and surgeon have the same magnification and the same field-of-view diameter of 22 mm. With a 125 mm binocular tube the magnification available to the surgeon will be lower and the field of view larger. This can be compensated if the surgeon uses, for instance, 12.5× eyepieces, and the co-observer a 10× eyepiece.

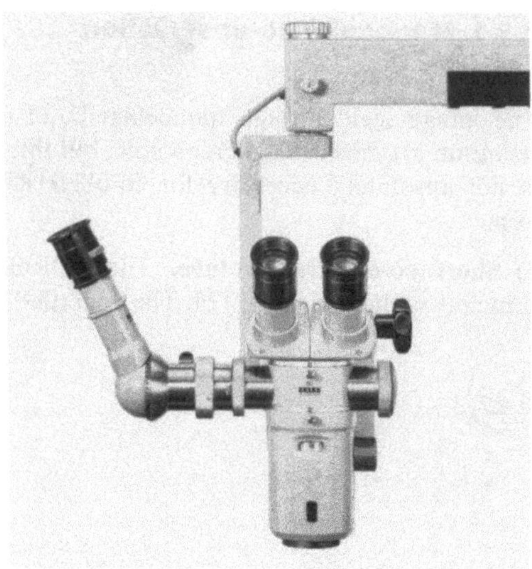

Fig. 130. Short co-observation tube on beam splitter side port.

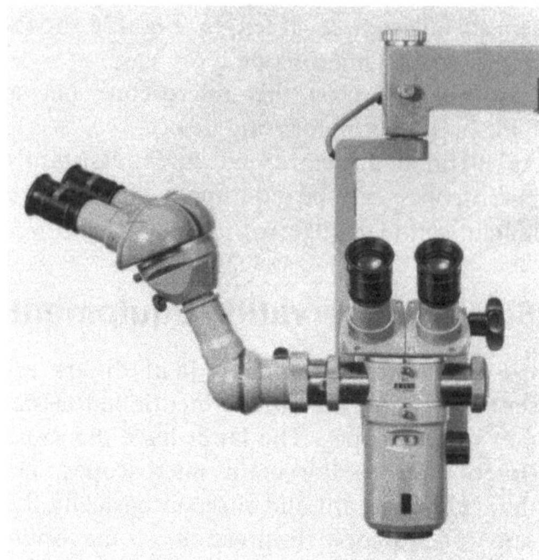

Fig. 131. Stereo co-observation tube.

Fig. 130 shows the co-observation tube with
a microscope. The tube length is 15 cm from
the point of rotation to the upper edge of the
eyepiece.

b) Long co-observation tube. If sterility must
be maintained and no interference with the
surgeon's work is allowed, the co-observation
tube must be longer for a longer distance
between co-observer and operating field.
The longer design requires a further intermediate image and thus a greater optical
outlay. A prism with two reflecting surfaces
in the tube's point of rotation reflects the
primary beam through 65°. The image rotation prism lies in the upper part of the 40 cm
long tube. Since the optical system has an
overall focal length of 160 mm, magnification and field-of-view diameter are the same
as mentioned in para. 6.3.1 a.

6.3.2 Stereo co-observation tube

Like the monocular co-observation tube the
stereo tube is fitted to one of the ports of the
beam splitter (Fig. 131). Stereoscopic observation is only possible with a binocular

tube with corresponding eyepieces. However,
due to the beam splitter only one of the
required observation beam paths is available. This may lead to the (false) assumption
that a binocular tube is used to view the
non-stereoscopic image only for more comfortable working like in optical microscopes
for histology. This is not the case because a
stereoscopic image is available thanks to
pupil splitting.

The principle of a stereo co-observation tube
can be explained, for instance, by an optical
microscope for histology if a binocular tube
is available. If one half of each of the exit
pupils behind the two eyepieces is occluded
by means of two diaphragms, the microscopic image will be three-dimensional. For
technical reasons the pupil splitting in the
stereo co-observation tube is not external
but internal. This is achieved by a splitting
prism in the parallel beam path. This prism
not only halves the pupils but also estab-
lishes an average distance of 22 mm between
the two primary rays; only then can a
binocular tube be used like on other operation and assistant's microscopes. While

operation microscopes and assistant's microscopes have a stereo basis of 22 mm (see para. 2.1.5) the stereo basis is here only ⅓ this value, i.e. 7 mm. This reduces the stereoscopic impression considerably, and a stereo co-observation tube is therefore well suited for stereoscopic co-observation but not for the cooperation of an assistant, for which it is too long. Its overall length is approx. 83 mm from the tube's point of rotation to the flange surface of the binocular tube. And last but not least the light loss is more than 50% compared with assistant's microscopes.

The stereo co-observation tube also contains an image rotation prism (in the mounting socket of the beam splitter) and a 65° deflecting prism. The 160 mm focal length of the tube objective again supplies magnifications and field-of-view diameters which correspond to those of the two monocular co-observation tubes.

7 Asepsis and methods of sterilization

Microscope manufacturers can neither supply methods of sterilization nor operation techniques with their instruments. As far as sterilization is concerned their responsibility is the delivery of clinically tested instruments and accessories such as sterilizable tubes or caps which are "tailor-made" for operation microscopes.

7.1 Sterility of operation microscopes

It is unavoidable that the surgeon touches or adjusts controls or even the entire microscope before and during surgical procedures. The corresponding controls or the complete instrument must therefore be sterile, and this can be realized by any of the following methods.

7.1.1 Instrument and accessories draped in sterile cloths for asepsis

Before an operation microscope, accessories, carrier arms, and stand column are completely enfolded in sterile cloths. This is a most reliable and economic method because the cloths can be repeatedly used when resterilized. Unfortunately certain operating controls, for instance, for magnification change and axial focusing are neither visible nor accessible under the cloths. The problem can be overcome by motorized magnification change and focusing. The difficulties encountered in adjusting the instrument can be avoided if sufficient space is provided under the covers.

Instead of in sterile cloths microscope and accessories can be draped in transparent, sterile plastic, a method which has proved its worth in many years of use. The microscope's operating controls remain visible under the plastic covers and are easier to operate. Both above-mentioned methods have one major drawback: the microscope illuminators produce heat which heats up the lamp housing to temperatures exceeding the operating temperature and shortens the life of the lamp. An additional ventilation system is necessary for the exhaust air.

7.1.2 Complete sterilization of the operation microscope

The entire microscope and its accessories are sterilized. The simplest method is to leave microscope and accessories on the carrier arms of the stand and drape them in plastic containing sterilization tablets. The equipment is sterilized overnight, and a few manipulations make it ready for operation the next day.

7.1.3 Microscope partially draped for asepsis

All operating elements used by the surgeon before and during the surgical procedure are provided with sterile caps and sleeves (7.2). This is obviously the best and most economic method, although it takes some time for the surgeon to indicate which controls he will need. If on the other hand the operation microscope must be frequently adjusted during surgery, and many different operating controls used this method is inconvenient and time-consuming.

7.1.4 Electrical controls

If all functions of microscope and accessories are foot- or hand-panel-controlled, sterilization is not absolutely necessary. The development of modern surgical techniques, for instance, in vitreous surgery, is marked by a trend towards electrical controls.

7.2 Sterilizable sleeves and caps

Fig. 132 shows a selection of sterilizable metal sleeves and rubber caps for operation microscopes and accessories. They can be sterilized like surgical instruments, by hot air, in autoclaves or by means of gas sterilization (see section 7.3). The rubber caps are subject to wear and tear become brittle and must be replaced after some time.

7.3 Methods of sterilization

Sleeves and caps can be sterilized like surgical instruments, for example,

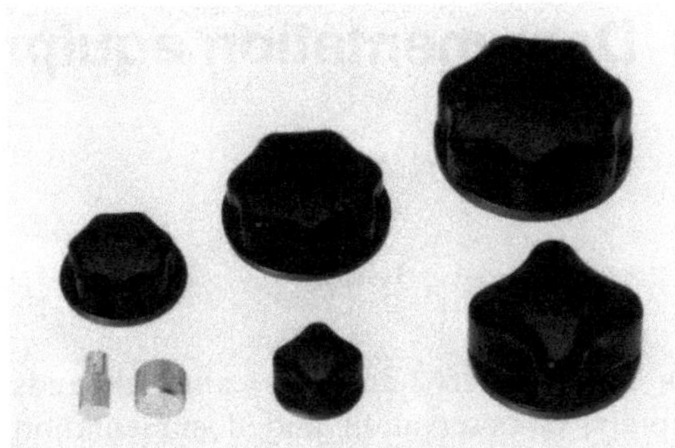

Fig. 132. Sterilizable sleeves and caps for operating controls of operation microscopes and accessories.

a) by hot air at 180 °C for one hour;
b) in an autoclave at 120 to 140 °C, 0.25 to 0.5 N/mm² for 10 minutes;
c) by gas sterilization for two hours according to the Sterivit method using a gas mixture of 15% ethlyen oxide and 85% carbonic acid at 45 °C, 60% sterilization humidity, and 0.55 N/mm².

Because of possible damage to optics and lacquer finish all other microscope modules cannot be subjected to the extreme conditions of the above-mentioned methods.

8 Documentation equipment

As microsurgery develops and expands rapidly, co-observation and documentation [1, 9b] facilities are becoming more and more important. The introduction of the beam splitter was a milestone in this development because this item allows attachments and accessories for co-observation and documentation to be subsequently fitted to microscopes already in use for several years. The change, for instance, from co-observation to still or cine photography becomes a matter of a few manipulations. Fig. 133 shows the beam splitter and some of the accessories it accommodates. Of the documentation methods for still and cine photography and TV recording, 35 mm photography is certainly the most popular. It requires only little instrument outlay to record the most important stages of microsurgical procedures. Depending on the chosen equipment, the surgeon can even control the exposures from a foot panel: cameras with automatic exposure control and automatic film transport guarantee superior results, and photography itself does not interfere with the surgical procedure. From a foot panel the surgeon can control the exposure of a series of color photographs to be taken of a surgical procedure, which he can later use for training and instruction.

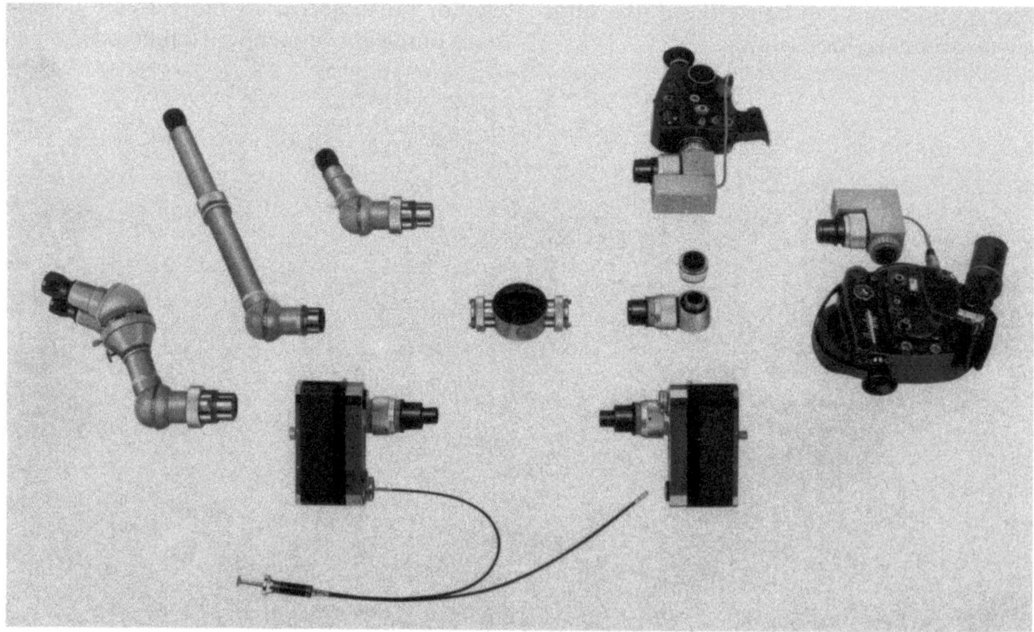

Fig. 133. Co-observation and documentation equipment which can be accommodated on the beam splitter.

Cine cameras document continuous dynamic processes and supply, for instance, a record of a complicated operation or instruction material for young surgeons. Subsequent sound recording by the surgeon is possible if he wants to comment on the operation technique he used. Although both formats – Super 8 and 16 mm – can be used, 16 mm films lend themselves especially for lectures, because of the higher image quality. Super 8 films are generally the choice for internal use. TV equipment is applied whenever co-observation of a large audience is wanted, especially to inform the team in the operating theater about state or progress of surgical treatment and perhaps comment on it, or to relay the events directly from the operating theater to any number of monitors in other rooms. Since video tape recording is also documentation in the narrower sense of the word, it is discussed here, too. Compared with cine photography video tape recording has some disadvantages and these are probably the reason why 16 mm films are preferred for lectures. First of all video tape recording requires great technical outlay, the reproduction of the image quality is not always satisfactory, and owing to the different TV standards compatible reproduction equipment for a specific type of video tape cannot be assumed to be available at international meetings or congresses. Video tape recording is, however, most valuable for training courses on microsurgery, because a microsurgical procedure stored on video tape is immediately available and can be shown to an audience any number of times.

General demands on documentation equipment

a) The device should be small, handy and lightweight, because it is mounted directly on the microscope and should not interfere with the latter's adjustment and operation.

b) A special adapter is required to accommodate the camera on the microscope. The optical system of the adapter adjusts the microscopic image to the required photo-graphic format. More sophisticated adapters also include manual or automatic diaphragm controls. All cine and TV cameras must have standard C mounts for direct connection to cine and TV adapters.

c) A pre-condition for the use of documentation equipment is adequate exposure of the film material and/or sufficient illumination of the TV camera tube. To achieve this, five different parameters must be coordinated:

I) Operation microscope or supplementary illuminator must be equipped with light sources of sufficient intensity. White light supplied, for instance, by halogen sources, is preferable. For cine or TV cameras the light sources must emit continuous radiation which is also required for observation by surgeon and assistant. Although attempts are made to use the same light sources also for photography, an electronic flash with a duration of only about 2/1000 s is preferable because it prevents blurring of the image. High-intensity light sources should not expose the operating field to excessive heat. With the exception of ophthalmic microsurgery, the use of an electronic flash is unproblematic. For cine photography, however, the operating field is exposed to intensive irradiation for quite some time, which should be reduced by a heat filter. Damage to the operating field can be avoided by flushing with salt solution.

II) The microscope magnification has only limited influence on correct exposure and illumination. First of all it must be such that the representation of a specific area of the operating field satisfies the surgeon. The same area should also be covered by the format of the documentation device used. In exceptional cases, for instance, in larynx photography, the dim light will require lower magnification so that a more or less extensive surrounding field is covered as well.

III) All adapters for documentation equipment contain an aperture stop to regulate the light intensity and at the same time adjust the depth of focus for the camera. If the intensity of the light source is high enough, and film material or TV camera tube are of high speed or sensitivity respectively, a small stop diameter (high f/number) will do, which guarantees great depth of focus. Focusing of the object field is then less critical.

IV) The exposure time as a setting parameter is variable within certain limits only for photography. The longest exposure time that is possible with continuous light emitters is exceeded if the operating field is blurred. A value determined through experience for ophthalmic microsurgery is 1/60 s. In other fields of surgery even 1/8 s may supply useful results. A series of test exposures at different exposure times is recommended to determine the most favorable exposure conditions for every type of instrument.

The exposure time for cine photography depends on the chosen exposure frequency which is 18 or 24 frames/s. In the case of subsequent sound recording only 24 frames/s can be used. The exposure time is irrelevant for TV recording. Differences are due to the TV standards (50 or 60 fields/s), but the determining factor is the sensitivity of the TV camera.

V) The demands on the light source and the above-mentioned exposure conditions are essentially determined by the speed of the photographic emulsion used in the documentation device. Quality and success of photography depend on it. Because of the higher information content only color films – color reversal films in particular – are used for still photography, since slides are generally the choice for training, instruction and lectures. Reversal film is even used if clichées are to be made of slides. Film with a fine grain is desirable. However, the finer the grain of the film the lower its speed, which contradicts the above statements, and requires the search for a compromise. Fortu-

nately there are high-speed films on the market with a grain which has no marked effect. Ektachrome High Speed Film, for instance, can be developed so as to gain about two f/numbers without considerably reducing the image quality.

Polaroid color photography is mentioned here merely for the sake of completeness; it has not found general acceptance because it does not fulfil the above-mentioned requirements. Because of the larger format Polaroid photography needs a much higher light intensity, and the removal of the photograph in the immediate vicinity of the operating field is certainly awkward. Instant photography lends itself, however, for courses.

8.1 Still photography

8.1.1 Illumination equipment

The general demands on documentation equipment [8 b] are listed in chapter 8. The details with respect to still photography are discussed below.

Two types of continuous emitters needed for observation, incandescent or halogen lamps, are also suited for still photography; the electronic flash is an alternative. Table 11 lists the advantages and disadvantages of both systems. It should be remembered that halogen lamps can also be used with fiber optics systems.

8.1.2 Photo adapters

As shown by the beam paths in Fig. 134, photo, cine, and TV adapters are of similar design and mounted on the operation microscope in similar ways. The beam splitter is inserted in the parallel beam path between magnification changer and binocular tube. The adapter is plugged into the lateral mounting piece and its position secured with a compression nut. Fig. 134 shows the photo

Table 11. Advantages and disadvantages of incandescent or halogen lamps and of an electronic flash as light sources for still photography

Incandescent or halogen lamp	Electronic flash
Advantages	*Advantages*
a) Adjustable, optimum object illumination	a) Higher intensity
b) Elimination of disturbing reflections by adjustment of the microscope's illumination system	b) High f/numbers
c) No limitation of the working distance	c) Greater depth of focus
d) Continuous emitter required for observation, also suitable for cine and TV	d) Less critical focusing on object details
	e) Short exposure times (some ms)
	f) No danger of blurring
	g) Higher magnifications because of higher intensity
Disadvantages	*Disadvantages*
a) Low intensity	a) No forecast of optimum illumination or disturbing reflections possible
b) Longer exposure times	b) Surgeon may be dazzled
c) Blurring of the image	c) Only usable for photography; additional incandescent or halogen lamp required for observation
d) Little depth of focus at high apertures (low f/numbers)	d) Higher technical outlay also for power supply of the flash
e) High magnifications almost impossible because of low depth of focus	e) Limited working distance

adapter $f = 220$ mm above, and the two cine adapters $f = 137$ mm and $f = 107$ mm below. According to the beam paths a positive lens element is required in every adapter to produce from the parallel light bundle an image of the desired format at a finite distance. The different formats of 35 mm film, TV camera tubes, 16 and 8 mm film require different focal lengths. To obtain a sharp image a circular, 22 mm dia. stop is provided in the photo adapter. If the entire format is to be utilized and if sufficient light is available, the stop should be replaced by a supplementary objective of 2× magnification.

a) Photo adapter. This is shown in Fig. 135. Its focal length is 220 mm, and the design principle corresponds to that shown in Fig. 134. An adapter ring is required to accommodate a 35 mm camera. For utilization of the entire 35 mm format (instead of a circular, 22 mm dia. area) a 2× supplementary objective is available for insertion between photo adapter and adapter ring. If a format larger than the 22 mm dia. image area is wanted but sufficient light is not available, the 1.6× supplementary objective is recommended instead of the 2× objective. The adapter has an adjustable f/number scale; the highest f/number is 64, the lowest 14.

b) Automatic photo adapter. Its design (Fig. 136) is similar to that of the adapter described in para. a) above. Its focal length is also 220 mm, and it also requires an adapter ring to accommodate the 35 mm

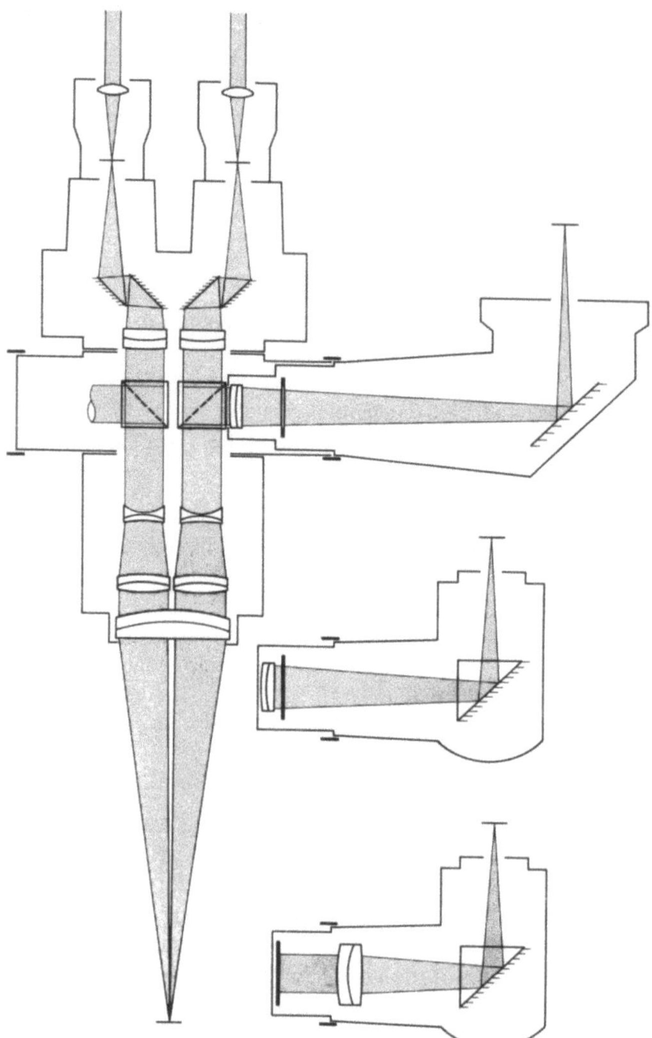

camera. A 2× supplementary objective must be inserted if the entire image format is to be utilized.

The automatic photo adapter automatically supplies correctly exposed photographs even with a simple cassette, although the use of 35 mm cameras with automatic film transport (spring mechanism, winder or motorized) is recommended. Whether or not the photographic system is draped in sterile cloths is then irrelevant. Furthermore, no additional personnel is required for photography and there is no interference with the time sequence of the operation. Only the film speed (25 to 400 ASA or 15 to 27 DIN) and the exposure time (between 1 and 1/30 s) have to be adjusted on the automatic photo adapter. Only about 10% of the light supplied to the adapter is required for exposure control. The integral measurement is made within an area of 12 mm dia. This area is doubled by a supplementary objective. The stop of the photo adapter is motorized and automatically adjusted to the

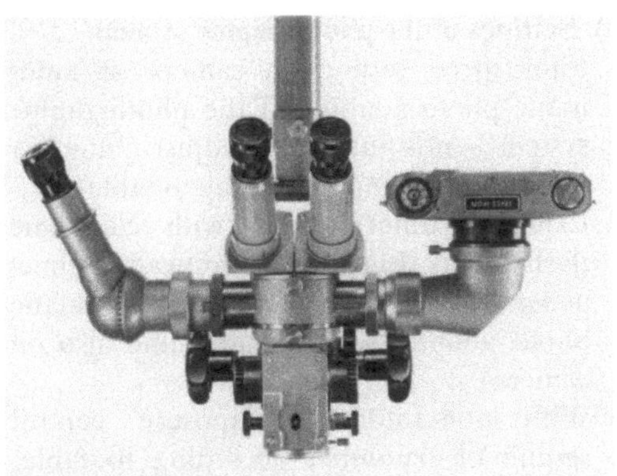

Fig. 135. Photo adapter $f = 220$ mm (right) and short co-observation tube (left).

f/numbers 14 to 64 within only 0.3 s. Acoustic signals indicate the two extreme positions of the stop, so that the light required for photography can be retained within the effective f/number range by suitable selection of the setting parameters lamp brightness, magnification, and exposure time.

The automatic photo adapter is powered by two batteries, each with a life of about two years. Their charge can be checked by means of a luminous diode. The batteries

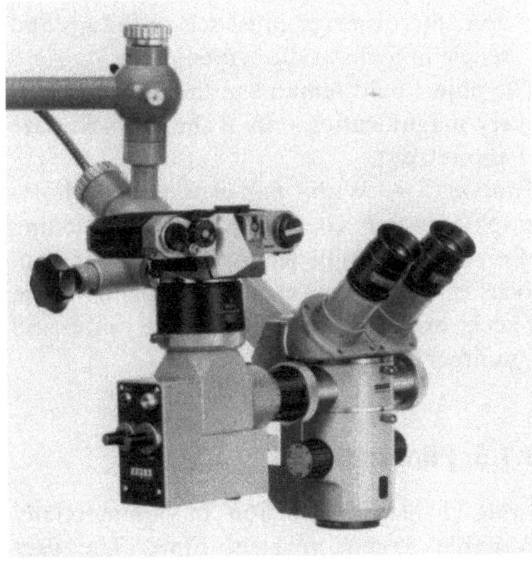

Fig. 136. Automatic photo adapter for operation microscopes.

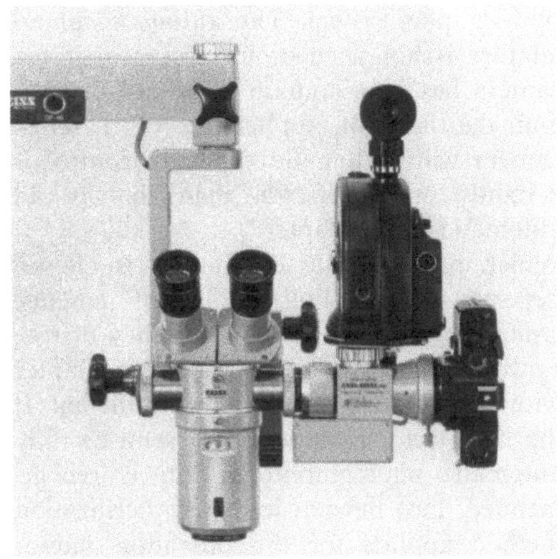

Fig. 137. Twin adapter (Urban) for the simultaneous mounting of a 35 mm camera and a TV camera.

are not necessary, for instance, on the motorized ceiling mount or on a mobile floor stand, because there the adapter is fed from the power supply of the stand.

c) Twin adapter. This is a special type of photo adapter to accommodate on one side of the beam splitter a 35 mm camera and (preferably) a compact TV camera simultaneously (Fig. 137). The adapter supplies the correct image format for both systems, i.e. it has two different focal lengths. A cube splits the beams for the two systems. The twin adapter has the great advantage that the opposite port of the beam splitter can be used for co-observation, for instance.

8.1.3 35 mm camera

The above-mentioned photo adapters accept all commercial 35 mm cameras from the simplest camera attachment to the most sophisticated professional reflex camera with automatic exposure control, motorized film transport, and IR-remote controlled release. There are simple criteria for the compilation of a technically and economically feasible photographic system. The automatic photo adapter is not needed, for instance, if the camera has an automatic exposure control, and the field of application of a reflex camera with automatic exposure control is certainly more versatile than that of an automatic photo adapter.

Which photographic equipment is chosen depends on the individual requirements. One basic criterion is the frequency of use. For occasional use the simple photo adapter with camera back may be quite sufficient. If the time factor is important a semi or fully automatic photographic system is recommended. Last but not least, the sterilization method applied for the operation microscope should be considered; if the whole instrument is draped in sterile cloths, an automatic photographic system with foot-panel-controlled camera release may be a necessity.

8.1.4 Photography

Some information is given here about the use of the photographic equipment, especially about the settings on photographic system and microscope.

a) Equipment of the operation microscope
1. Beam splitter for accommodation of the photo adapter (preferably beam splitter 70).
2. Photo adapter 220 mm or automatic photo adapter.
3. Adapter ring (depending on the camera type).
4. Supplementary objective 1.6 or 2× (without supplementary objective the 30° funnel stop must be inserted in the camera housing to define the image format).
5. 35 mm camera.
6. Camera release.
7. Reticle in one of the two eyepieces.
8. Electronic flash (if the available light is insufficient and the exposure time therefore too long).

b) Settings of the photographic system
1. Film speed setting on camera or automatic photo adapter (if the photographic system is not automatic, adjust f/number and exposure time according to table).
2. Exposure time: 1/30 s (with electronic flash set to shutter synchronization time, generally 1/50 to 1/60 s); with automatic photo adapter set exposure time also on camera.
3. With non-automatic exposure control setting of f/number according to table; with automatic photo adapter or automatic camera the f/number is automatically set.
4. Exposure.
5. Film transport (unless the camera is motorized).

c) Settings of the microscope
1. Eyepiece adjustment so that the reticle is in focus for the observer; important: always turn from + to −.
2. *PD* setting on binocular tube.
3. Adjustment of microscope to working position.
4. Focusing on the object field at low magnification, followed by parallax-free focusing on the specimen at maximum magnification; the observer must see specimen and reticle in focus at the same time.

The object field remains in the focal plane at every magnification only if the eyepieces are at about 0 dpt.

Caution! – With non-automatic photographic system check the f/number setting after magnification change. If the depth of focus is insufficient, use lower magnification. Check exposure data (exposure time and f/number) again.

8.1.5 Film material

Table 12 lists a selection of commercially available 35 mm reversal films. The user may, of course, also use other film materials for test exposures.

Table 12. 35 mm reversal films

Film type	Film speed DIN/ASA	Cartridge	Artificial light	Daylight filter	No. of exposures
Agfa-Gevaert					
Agfachrome 50 S Prof.	18/50	135 – 36		×	36
Agfachrome 50 L Prof.	18/50	135 – 36	×		36
Agfacolor 80 S Prof.	20/80	135 – 36		×	36
Fuji					
Fujichrome R 100	21/100	135 – 24		×	24
		135 – 36		×	36
Kodak					
High-speed Ektachrome EH	23/160	135 – 36		×	36
		135 – 20		×	20
High-speed Ektachrome B/EHB	22/125	135 – 36	×		36
		135 – 20	×		20

8.1.6 Frequently used formulae

Only the formulae relating to magnification and object field are listed below. Further formulae for the determination of resolving power, depth of focus, etc. are given in chapter 10.

a) Magnification referred to the film plane. For 35 mm photography with $f_{Ad} = 220$ mm photo adapter the magnification in the film plane is calculated according to the formula

$$M_F = \frac{f_{Ad}}{f_O} \gamma,$$

where f_{Ad} is the focal length of the adapter (here 220 mm), f_O the focal length of the microscope objective, and γ the magnification factor of the operation microscope's 5-stage or zoom magnification changer (the values of γ are listed in Table 2).

Numerical example

If the focal length of the microscope objective f_O is 200 mm, that of the photo adapter $f_{Ad} = 220$ mm, and the magnification factor $\gamma = 1.6$ (corresponding to position 25 of the 5-stage magnification changer), the magnification $M_F = (220/200) \cdot 1.6 = 1.76$. The image of the circular operating field produced in the film plane will thus be $1.76 \times$ enlarged. A funnel stop of 22 mm dia. must be inserted in the camera for a focused image, but then the 35 mm format cannot be fully utilized. This can be avoided by a $2 \times$ supplementary objective between photo adapter and camera adapter ring. The magnification will then be

$$M_F = \frac{2f_{Ad}}{f_O} \gamma.$$

With the above values and $2 \times$ supplementary objective the magnification in the film plane is $M_F = 3.52$.

b) Dimensions of the object field. Besides the magnification referred to the film plane the dimensions of the object field on the film may be of interest. The simplest method to determine them is by a sterile scale next to the object area which is photographed together with the operating field. Independent of the re-enlargement of the negative the feature of interest can always be determined by means of the photographed scale.

The object field covered by an image can, of course, also be determined by means of the instrument data. Without the above-mentioned supplementary objective and after calculation of the magnification M_F the diameter of the circular object field is 22 mm/M_F. If, according to the above example, $M_F = 1.76$ the diameter of the object field is 12.5 mm, provided the inserted stop has a diameter of 22 mm.

The 35 mm format is fully utilized with $2\times$ supplementary objective and without 22 mm stop. The object field M_O is then

$$M_O = \frac{24\,\text{mm}}{M_F} \cdot \frac{36\,\text{mm}}{M_F} .$$

According to the above-mentioned numerical example the magnification with supplementary objective $M_F = 3.52$, is therefore approximately 6.8×10.2 mm.

Such considerations and calculations are too tedious and time-consuming for practical work, for which a reticle with a rectangle in one of the two eyepieces is recommended. Features within this rectangle are covered by the 35 mm format with supplementary objective.

8.2 Cine photography

As mentioned above, Super 8 and particularly 16 mm films are becoming more and more important for instruction and lectures. Their advantages are brilliant reproduction of the surgical procedure, unproblematic, automatic photography, and suitable projection facilities for 16 mm film at meetings and congresses. Cine photography is more expensive than still photography but an indispensable piece of equipment for showing dynamic processes such as surgical procedures.

8.2.1 Illumination systems

Only continuous emitters can be used, i.e. incandescent and preferably halogen lamps, the latter either built in (operation microscopes of the H type) or in combination with a fiber optics system. Older microscope types have only incandescent lamps, which must be run at overload during cine photography for reasons of light intensity and color temperature. A fiber optics system improves the exposure conditions also of older illumination systems.

8.2.2 Cine adapter and cine cameras

As seen in Fig. 134, para. 8.1.2, photo and cine adapters are of similar design. First of all the adapter connects the cine camera opto-mechanically with the beam splitter. Since they are attached to the side port of the beam splitter, a positive lens element of suitable focal length must produce from the parallel beam path which leaves the beam splitter an image covering the format at a finite distance. Adapter focal lengths of 74 mm and 137 mm are required for Super 8 or 16 mm film respectively. Another adapter with a focal length of 107 mm is available for 16 mm film, which is recommended for critical light conditions, e.g. for cine photography of the larynx through the microscope.

All cine adapters are provided with an adjustable diaphragm. Adjustment is made by means of a ring with engraved f/numbers from 7 to 32 for the 74 mm cine adapter, and from 8 to 44 for the 137 mm cine adapter. The diaphragm adjustment of older cine adapters must be done manually, that of the latest models is done automatically by means of a motorized diaphragm setting mechanism which is controlled by a sensor in the cine camera.

The automatic diaphragm control is most important for practical work, because it guarantees optimally exposed films under all illumination conditions of the operating field. It should be remembered in this connection that for given microscope equipment

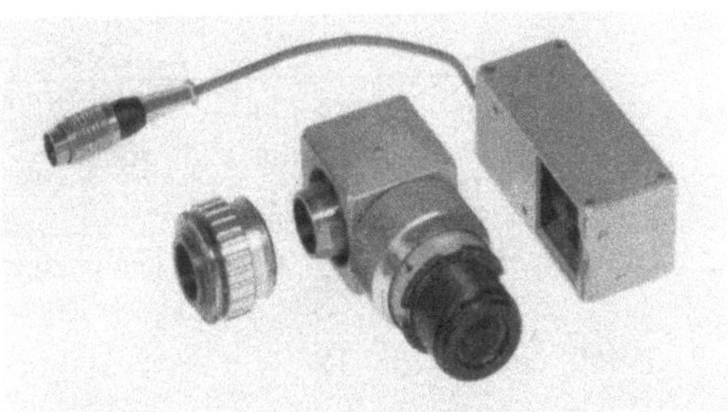

Fig. 138. Design of cine adapters with automatic diaphragm control.

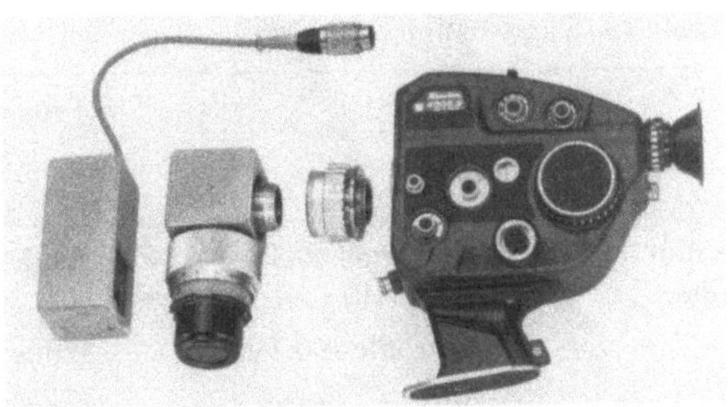

Fig. 139. Automatic diaphragm control and Beaulieu Super 8 camera "4008-S-Zeiss".

the light available for exposure of the film depends not only on the reflection conditions of the operating field itself, but also on the magnification set. This means that the diaphragm must be re-adjusted whenever the magnification changer is operated. Without automatic exposure control and automatic diaphragm adjustment this is a tedious and time-consuming process, which will supply satisfactory results only after long experience.

All three cine adapters are of the same design regarding the automatic diaphragm drive. As shown in Fig. 138 they comprise from left to right the adapter piece with standard C mount, the cine adapter with a focal length of 74, 107 or 137 mm, and the diaphragm drive with connecting cable. The sensor for the automatic diaphragm control of the cine adapters is contained in the cine camera. Via a control loop it controls the motor for the correct diaphragm setting. The regulating system takes into consideration the film speed (from 10 to 400 ASA or 11 to 27 DIN) and the number of frames per second (2 to 70). Cine camera, control loop and diaphragm drive are fed from a chargeable NiCd battery.

For the above-mentioned reasons specially designed "Beaulieu" cameras are required, which are available under the designations "R 16 Zeiss" and/or "4008 S-Zeiss". Fig. 139 shows the "4008 S-Zeiss" with diaphragm drive, 74 mm cine adapter and adapter ring

with standard C mount, and "Beaulieu" Super 8 camera. Figs. 88 and 137 show the "Beaulieu" camera with automatic diaphragm drive on a zoom microscope.

The "Urban" cine camera (Fig. 140) for 16 mm film has met with considerable approval among experts owing to its small dimensions and low weight. Easy interchangeability of the cassette is another important feature of this camera. For long operations a 60 m film spool which would unnecessarily load microscope and mounting is not required, but only two easily exchangeable cassettes.

The "Urban" cine camera cannot be used with the automatic cine adapter with auto-

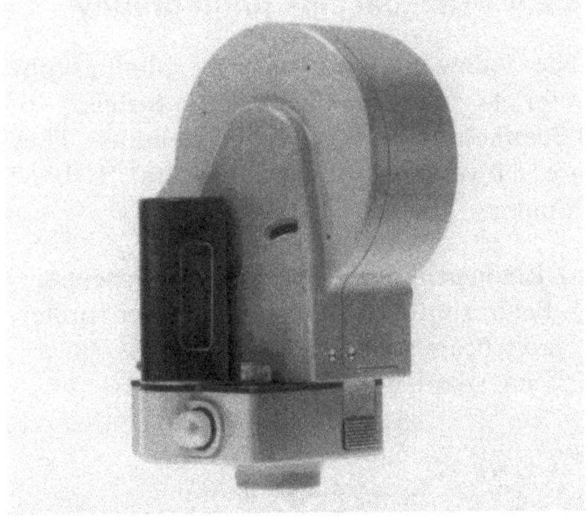

Fig. 140. 16 mm Urban cine camera.

Table 13. 8 and 16 mm color films

	Film type	Type of light	Film speed		Length of film [m]	Perfora-tion
			ASA	DIN		
8 mm film	Kodachrome 40 Type A (KMA 464P)	artificial	40	17	15	
	Ektachrome 160 Type A	artificial	160	23	15	
16 mm film	Kodachrome 40 Type A (KMA 464P)	artificial	40	17	30/120	one-or
	Ektachrome 160 Type A	artificial	160	23	30/120	twosided

matic diaphragm drive. In all other respects the cine adapter corresponds to the above-mentioned 107 or 137 mm automatic cine adapters. The "Urban" cine camera is only for 18 frames/s. The corresponding film material, perforated on one side, is commercially available.

8.2.3 Film material

Table 13 lists film material that is most frequently used for documentation in microsurgery. This is only a small selection of the many available film types. The user himself will eventually decide which suits his purposes best.

8.2.4 Practical cine photography

The following hints for cine photography refer to the "Beaulieu 4008 S-Zeiss" or "Beaulieu R 16-Zeiss" cine cameras. They are, however, also valid for the "Urban" camera.

a) Equipment of the operation microscope.
1. Beam splitter for the cine adapter (preferably beam splitter 70).
2. Cine adapter.
3. Adapter ring with C mount.
4. Diaphragm drive.
5. Cine camera.
6. Wire release.
7. Battery handle.
8. Reticle in one of the two eyepieces.
9. Supplementary illuminator, if necessary.

b) Settings on the cine equipment
1. Set film speed on camera.
2. Set frame frequency.
3. Connect diaphragm drive cable to cine camera.
4. Exposure.

c) Settings on the microscope
1. Adjust eyepieces so that the observer sees the reticle in focus. *Important:* always turn from + to −.
2. Adjust *PD* on binocular tube.
3. Adjust microscope to working position.
4. Focus on the operating field at low magnification, then focus parallax-free on the specimen at highest magnification. The observer must see specimen and reticle in focus at the same time. The object field will remain in the focal plane at every magnification only if the eyepieces are set to a value near approx. 0 dpt. Adjust desired magnification.

9 Maintenance of the operation microscope

An operation microscope comprises in the widest sense of the word the microscope, the couplings, carrier arms, stands with electrical power supply, and accessories for assistants, co-observation and documentation. Depending on the frequency of its use, a service technician should carry out a complete service at least every 5 years. Besides this regular service the following hints should be followed.

Clean lacquered surfaces only with a clean, soft brush or cloth. For contaminated surfaces use benzine, never acetone or ether.

Cover the microscope when not in use. Never leave the microscope without objective, binocular tube and eyepieces. Keep accessories, and especially objectives, tubes and eyepieces which are not needed in dust-proof containers.

Wipe off blood splashes, detergent spots or bone splinters on the microscope with a soft cloth soaked in a surface-active, luke-warm detergent. This applies in particular to splashes of salt solution on the objective. If they are not removed immediately after surgery, they form a film which destroys the anti-reflection coating.

Contaminated optical surfaces cause stray-light which in turn reduces the contrast. However, clean only the outer surfaces of objectives and eyepieces. Remove dust with a rubber ball or a grease-free brush (rinse in ether before use). Wipe off fingerprints and similar contaminations with a cotton wad soaked in acetone on a wooden stick. All gliding surfaces, e.g. the focusing guides should be re-greased after extended use. This should be carried out by the maintenance service, who should also check whether the instrument complies with all safety regulations.

10 Formulae

10.1 Optical properties of operation microscopes

10.1.1 Magnification

The term magnification describes the size of an object viewed with unaided eye in comparison with that seen through an optical system [4].

A standard distance must be stipulated for observation with the unaided eye to be able to come to a generally valid comparison. 250 mm distance of clear vision have been agreed upon. The observed object is seen actual size if it is brought into the focal point of a lens or multi-element optical system with the focal length $f = 250$ mm and viewed with relaxed eye (without accommodation). Shorter focal lengths enlarge the image and vice versa.

The magnification is defined as

$$V = \frac{250}{f} \quad (f \text{ in mm}).$$

The equation contains a problem insofar as the distance of clear vision is coupled with the eye's capacity of accommodation, and weakens with increasing age. The value 250 mm is valid for middle age, it then increases, and the magnification of the optical system rises perceptibly.

With the above information the magnification of an operation microscope can be easily determined.

The microscope consists of a primary objective (f_O), a tube lens (f_T), an eyepiece (f_E); and a magnification changer or zoom system with different telescope magnifications (γ) which can be arranged between primary objective and tube lens.

It follows for the magnification of the individual optical elements that $V_O = 250/f_O$, $V_T = f_T/250$ (for f_O the parallel beam path runs against the direction of the light), $V_E = 250/f_E$. γ is set for the Galilean magnification changer or zoom system. The result of multiplication of these terms is the total magnification of an operation microscope

$$V_M = \frac{f_T}{f_O} \cdot \gamma \cdot V_E.$$

In the case of documentation, cine or TV, the magnification is referred to as image scale M_F which is determined according to the formula

$$M_F = \frac{f_A}{f_O} \cdot \gamma,$$

where f_A is the focal length of the photo or cine adapter.

10.1.2 Object fields

The size of an imaged object field is limited by the size of the field-of-view diaphragm in the eyepiece or by the photographic or cine format. The image scale of object to field-of-view diaphragm or film plane is the decisive parameter. All eyepieces for Zeiss operation microscopes have the same product of field-of-view diameter (S_E) and eyepiece magnification ($S_E \cdot V_E = 200$). It follows for the object-field diameter S_M of the microscope that

$$S_M = \frac{200}{V_M} \text{ [mm]}.$$

For documentation purposes Zeiss operation microscopes have the same angular field for all adapters. The adapter focal lengths are adapted to the different formats.

Consequently the object field of a specific combination of primary objective and magnification changer or zoom system has a constant diameter independent of the adapter focal length, to which the following equation applies:

$$S_F = \frac{f_O}{10 \cdot \gamma}.$$

With a combination photo adapter/Polaroid adapter, for instance, the object field of both pictures is of the same size.

10.1.3 Numerical aperture

It has been known since Ernst Abbe that detail recognition is not dependent upon the magnification alone. According to the diffraction theory the resolution of an optical system is determined by the numerical aperture, abbreviated N.A., which is the product of the refractive index of the medium surrounding the object and the sine of half the aperture angle.

High resolution therefore calls for high apertures, which, however, result in less depth of field. As this is inconsistent with the demand for a great depth of field for manipulations, a compromise must be found.

An equation can be derived for the numerical aperture, which combines mechanical and optical characteristics of an operation microscope. Because small aperture angles u allow the use of the sine instead of the tangent, it follows for the object-side aperture N.A. in air that

$$N.A. = \frac{\varnothing}{2f_O}$$

where f_O is the focal length of the objective and $\varnothing$ the aperture of the magnification changer or zoom system.

10.1.4 Graphic representation of the most important data (nomogram N1)

The many possible combinations of primary objective, magnification changer positions, tube lenses and eyepieces result in a great number of total magnifications and image scales. The total magnification V_M and the image scale M_F of an operation microscope can be taken from the nomogram; the object-field diameter S_M or S_F is also given.

The different focal lengths of the primary objective f_O can be found on the abscissa in the oblique rectangle in the center of the nomogram. The magnification γ of the Galilean changer or zoom system is plotted on the ordinate, and the points of intersection give the object-side apertures N.A.

The following is an example of visual observation. For an operation microscope with a primary objective $f_O = 400$, a tube $f_T = 125$, 10× eyepieces and changer position $\gamma = 3.2$, start at the point $f_O = 400$ and follow the arrow to the straight line through the point $\gamma = 3.2$ parallel to the abscissa. The corresponding object-side aperture N.A. is 0.02. To the right one reaches the vertical straight line $f_T = 125$ and 10×, where one reads off the value $V_M = 10$. The corresponding object field S_M has a diameter of 20 mm. For $f_T = 160$ and 20× eyepieces instead of $f_T = 125$ and 10× eyepieces, follow the horizontal line further to the right to the scale V_M where the value 26 is found with a corresponding diameter of the object field S_M of 7.8 mm.

The next example applies to documentation. For $f_O = 200$ and $\gamma = 0.63$ the numerical aperture N.A. = 0.025. Going from this point horizontally to the left leads to the object-field diameter $S_F = 32$ mm, and further to the left to $f_A = 220$ mm (photo adapter), for instance, and following the sloped line to the lower left to the image scale M_F leads to the value 0.7. With the same values of f_O and γ but a Polaroid adapter with $f_A = 700$ instead of the photo adapter, follow the horizontal

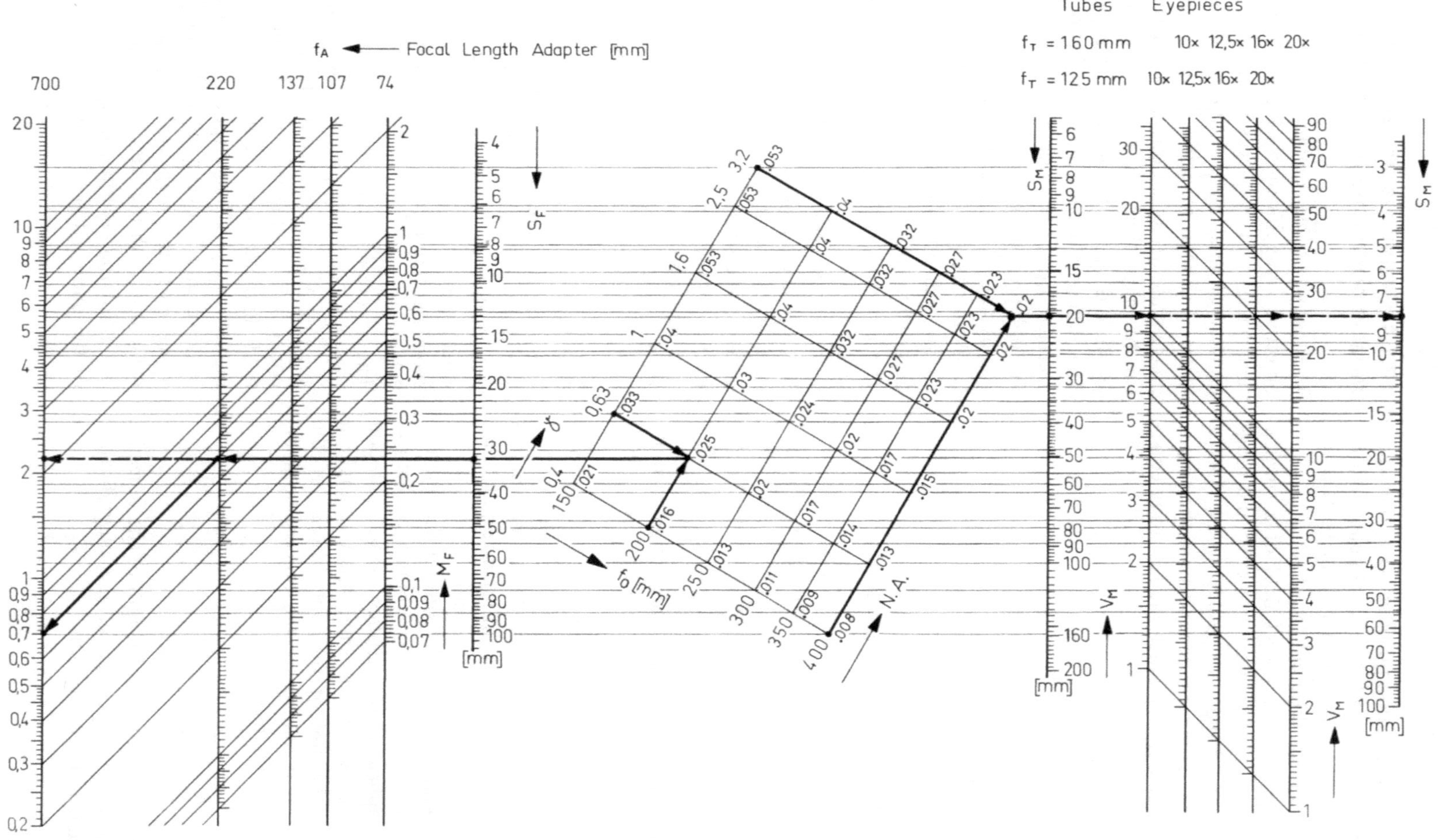

Documentation
Visual View
Tubes   Eyepieces
$f_T = 160$ mm   10x 12,5x 16x 20x
$f_T = 125$ mm   10x 12,5x 16x 20x
f_A — Focal Length Adapter [mm]
700   220   137 107   74
S_F
M_F
f_0 [mm]
N.A.
S_M
V_M
Nomogram N1

(dotted) line to the vertical line $f_A = 700$, which coincides with the scale M_F. The value $M_F = 2.2$ is obtained. Note that independent of the adapter, S_F is constant with given values of f_O and γ, because the angular field is the same for all adapters.

10.2 Detector properties

Visual observation is dependent upon the properties of the eye, documentation on those of the film.

10.2.1 Observation

The properties of the eye have been described in many publications, by Schober [11] for instance, but only relevant ones are considered here. Important parameters for resolving power and depth of focus are derived from the structure of the retina. The physiological angular resolving power has values between one and four angular minutes, i.e. punctiform features which the observer sees under this angle are still recognized.

A lower value applies to the recognizability of fine lines and fibrous features. The corresponding vernier visual acuity lies between five and ten angular seconds.

The depth of the receptors, which amounts to about 0.06 mm, results in an image space to which a certain object space is assigned by the optical system.

Another important property is the capacity of accommodation. It is dependent upon the observer's age and may have values between 8 and 0 diopters, i.e. a child is capable of seeing objects sharp which are up to 125 mm away, while this capacity is lost in old age.

10.2.2 Documentation

The film properties are dependent upon the structure of the photographic emulsion, a parameter which is also referred to as "grain size". The graininess of an exposed film is due to the accumulation of silver bromide grains. As a rule of thumb their diameter is determined by the division of the image diagonal by 1000.

10.3 Terms of the diffraction theory

Which depth of focus or resolving power is obtainable with an operation microscope can only be determined with the diffraction theory.

10.3.1 Airy disk

Not even an optical system without image aberrations images a point as a point, but as an intensity distribution known as Airy distribution. The point degenerates to a disk which is surrounded by a system of concentric rings, but owing to the intensity distribution only the first ring is generally clearly visible. The diameter of the Airy disk is determined by the following equation:

$$\varnothing_A = \frac{1.22\,\lambda}{\text{N.A.}}$$

where λ is the wavelength and N.A. the numerical aperture. For the sizing of an Airy disk restriction to the wavelength $\lambda = 550$ nm is sufficient for visual observation, because the spectral sensitivity of the light-adapted eye has its maximum around this wavelength.

The spectral sensitivity of the film material must be considered in case of unsharpness due to diffraction in photography (see section 10.5).

10.3.2 Limit of resolution

The limit of resolution of an optical system can now be determined. If illumination and observation apertures are almost equal – which is generally the case in operation

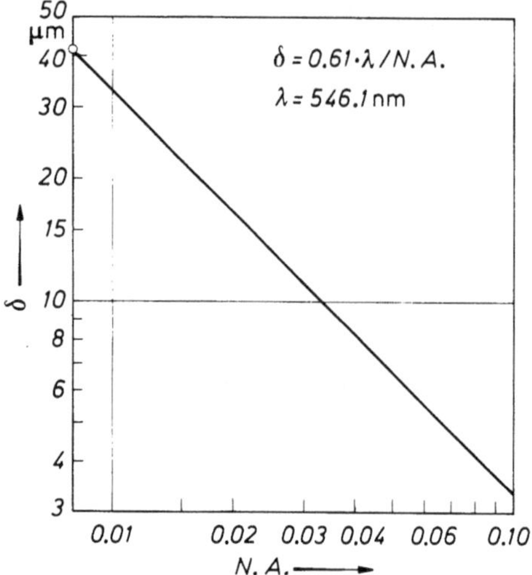

Fig. 141. Limit of resolution.

microscopes – it follows that according to the diffraction theory two bright spots on a black background can still be resolved if the distance between the centers of both Airy disks equals their radius. It then follows that

$$\delta = 1/2 \, \varnothing_A = \frac{0.61 \, \lambda}{\text{N. A.}}.$$

According to the graphic representation of this equation (Fig. 141) $\delta = 13.3 \, \mu$m for N.A. $= 0.025$.

10.3.3 Axial extension of the diffraction pattern

The axial spatial extension of an Airy disk is particularly important for an assessment of the depth of field. The axial depth of focus of the principal maximum d is given by the equation

$$d = \frac{4 \, \lambda}{(\text{N. A.})^2}.$$

According to Berek [3a, 3b] the average eighth, that is

$$d_D = \frac{\lambda}{2 \, (\text{N. A.})^2}$$

corresponds to a defocusing still recognizable by the observer.

10.4 Useful magnification

Two apparently independent parameters, magnification and numerical aperture are combined by this term. According to the equation

$$\varnothing_A = 2 f \tan w'$$

a system with a focal length f sees half the diameter of the Airy disk under an angular field w'. The focal length can be substituted by the magnification, which results in the equation

$$V = \frac{\tan w'}{\lambda} \, 500 \, (\text{N. A.})$$

where $\tan w'$ can be substituted by the physiological angular resolving power of 2 or 4 angular minutes, which results in the following relation given already by Abbe:

$$500 \, (\text{N.A.}) \leqq V \leqq 1000 \, (\text{N.A.})$$

This is the range of useful magnification, and the theoretical resolving power can be achieved within this range.

Within the range of useful magnification the exit pupils have diameters between 0.5 and 1 mm. If aperture or magnification is unknown, the exit pupils indicate whether an instrument works within the range of useful magnification.

Pupils below 0.5 mm lead to overmagnification, which is of advantage for measurement and counting, although the image is dark and entoptic phenomena interfere. More information is not obtainable. Pupil diameters above 1 mm result in undermagnification. The resolving power cannot be fully utilized, although the image is brighter, which may sometimes be of advantage.

10.5 Useful *f*/number

A comparison of the permissible circle of confusion with the diameter of the Airy disk results in a certain *f*/number K_C at which the unsharpness due to diffraction remains just invisible. It follows for U as diameter of the permissible circle of confusion that

$$U = \varnothing_A$$

For $\lambda = 550$ nm and $K = 1/2$ (N.A.) it follows that $K_C = 750 \cdot U$. For 35 mm film $U = 0.05$ mm, and consequently $K_C = 37.5$. For cine film $U = 0.015$ mm, and consequently $K_C = 11.3$. For large formats, e.g. Polaroid 90×120 mm $U = 0.1$, and consequently $K_C = 75$.

f/numbers above K_C result in unsharpness of the image due to diffraction (see section 10.6).

10.6 Depth of focus

10.6.1 Visual observation

The term depth of focus is well known from photography, for which it is unambiguously defined. Film material has the properties mentioned above, and the film plane has a fixed position with respect to the imaging optical system.

The conditions are different in visual observation, where the individual properties of the observer's eye are of decisive influence, i.e. a certain depth of focus applies only to the normal eye. Different formulae are given in the relevant literature for the calculation of the depth of focus.

One term of the depth of focus results from the diffraction theory, and a second term considers the properties of the eye. A third term which contains the accommodation must be added for observation without micrometer eyepiece.

The corresponding equation is as follows:

$$D F = \frac{\lambda}{(\text{N.A.})^2}\, c_1 + \frac{250}{V\,(\text{N.A.})}\, c_2$$
$$+ \frac{250^2}{V^2}\left(\frac{1}{S_N} - \frac{1}{S_F}\right)$$

where S_N is the distance of the near point and S_F the distance of the far point from the eye. The difference is the accommodation range.

According to Françon [5] c_1 has the value 1 if the significant axial extension of the Airy disk is assumed to be $\lambda/(\text{N.A.})^2$

He substitutes for c_2 the value $2'$ for the physiological angular resolving power.

According to [3 a] Berek found the constants $c_1 = \frac{1}{2}$ and $c_2 = 4.7'$ by measurement.

Measurements show that the formula Berek found under different conditions (higher total magnification and aperture) is also applicable to operation microscopes. It indicates the conditions better than Françon's equation, for example. Especially at low magnifications ($< 8\times$), which are possible with an operation microscope, the Airy disk can hardly be resolved, and the influence of the diffraction on the depth of focus becomes irrelevant. Berek's equation is better adapted to these conditions. He also mentions the term standard magnification, that is the magnification at which the apparent size of the Airy disk recognized by the eye corresponds to the limiting resolving power of the human eye. $\lambda = 0.55\ \mu$m and $1'$ result in a standard magnification of $160 \times$ N.A. The lowest magnifications of Zeiss operation microscopes are within this range.

Fig. 142 shows the normalized depth-of-focus curves according to Françon and Berek. The product of depth of focus DF and the square of the numerical aperture is plotted on the ordinate, the quotient of magnification and numerical aperture on the abscissa.

The run of both curves is similar in the range of useful magnification ($500 \leqq C \leqq 1000$), while it is different for $C < 500$.

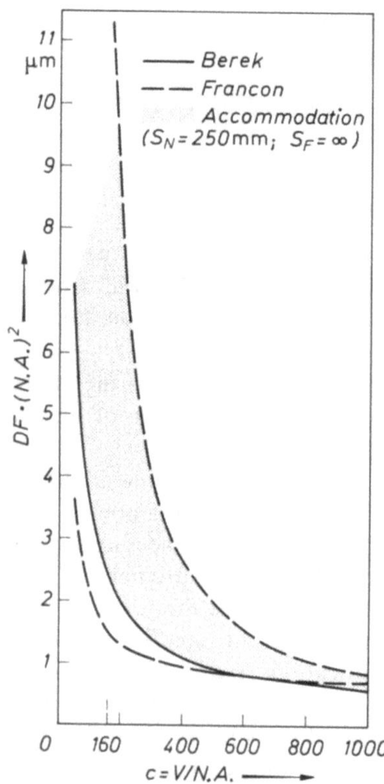

Fig. 142. Depth of field.

The hatched area is the range of accommodation (infinity to 4 diopters) of a middle-aged observer. The values are considerable for low magnifications. Considering that according to Schober accommodation from 0 (object at infinity) to 4 diopters is made within 0.8 s, the depth of focus is in some respects considerable.

The nomogram N2 is better suited for practical applications. The depth of focus DF in mm is plotted on the abscissa, while the first column of the ordinate lists the total magnification V_M, and the second column the accommodation range DF_{Acc}. DF and DF_{Acc} yield the total depth of focus. This leads to useful practical hints. According to the nomogram N2, the same total magnification is obtainable with different apertures by different combinations of the individual optical

elements. The depth of focus varies considerably as a function of the aperture. $V_M = 5.0$, for instance, results in values of DF between 2.4 and 13 mm.

This range can be considerably expanded by a depth of focus dependent upon the accommodation (see nomogram N2). The optimum combination can be found a certain depth of the operating field and a required detail recognition.

10.6.2 Documentation

The depth of focus for still and cine photography is determined according to the standard values of the permissible circle of confusion. Different values are given for the different formats. It is assumed that, depending on the format, re-enlargement of the picture is different, so that the circle of confusion U is no longer resolved by the eye. As mentioned in section 10.5 already, the following values apply:

35 mm format:	$U = 0.05$ mm
Normal 8, Super 8, 16 mm film:	$U = 0.015$ mm
Large format:	$U = 0.1$ mm

The following equation holds for the calculation of the depth of focus for documentation (DF_D):

$$D F_D = 2\,U \cdot \frac{K}{M_F^2} \; (K \leq K_C)$$

where M_F is the image scale from object to film plane and K the f/number which is determined from the focal length of the adapter f_A and the bundle diameter $\varnothing$ effective before the adapter, which is dependent upon the position of the magnification changer or zoom system. The f/number can be varied by an iris diaphragm with the diameter $\varnothing_I$ before the adapter which limits the aperture.

It generally applies that

$$K = K_{min}.$$
$$\varnothing_I = \varnothing$$

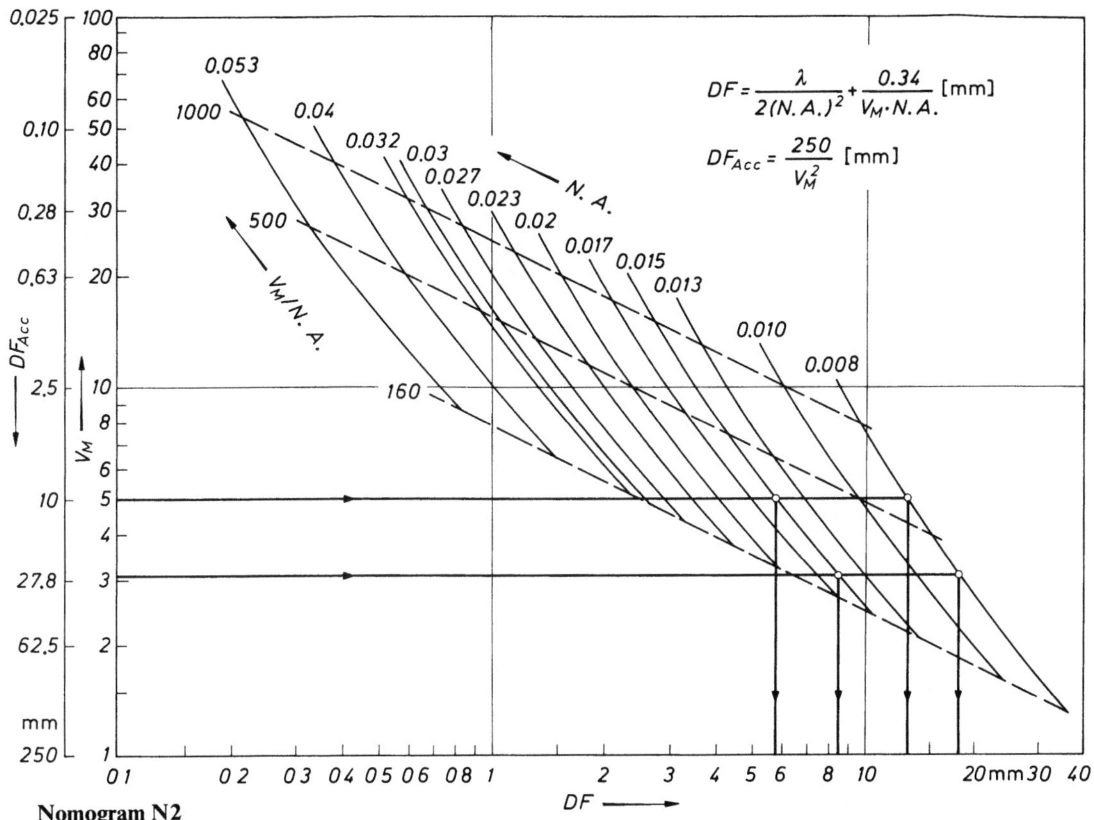

Nomogram N2

The numerical aperture of an instrument is then fully utilized and optimum resolution achieved. With $K > K_{min}$ ($\varnothing_I < \varnothing$) the resolution is lower, a measure taken to increase the depth of focus.

35 mm film and cinematography are most frequently used with operation microscopes, and are therefore the only ones considered here.

Unsharpness due to diffraction influences the depth of focus in photography and cinematography. Other than in amateur photography it is possible to stop down considerably, which leads to high f/numbers above the useful f/number indicated further above. In this case the Airy disks are larger than the circle of confusion. The diameter of the Airy disk must be taken to determine the depth of focus. It follows for the depth of focus that

$$D F_D = \frac{K^2}{375\, M_F^2}\ (K \geqq K_C).$$

The depth of focus can be determined using the nomograms N3, N4, and N5. The image scale M_F is plotted on the ordinate, the depth of focus DF_D in mm on the abscissa. Besides the curves of the f/numbers K the nomograms N3 to N5 also show the curves γ of magnification changer or zoom system, and the adapter curves f_A. The above-mentioned f/number K_{min} can be taken from the point of intersection of these three curves. The depth of focus is determined by means of two examples.

An operation microscope consists of a primary objective $f_O = 200$ mm and a Galilean magnification changer in position $\gamma = 0.4$.

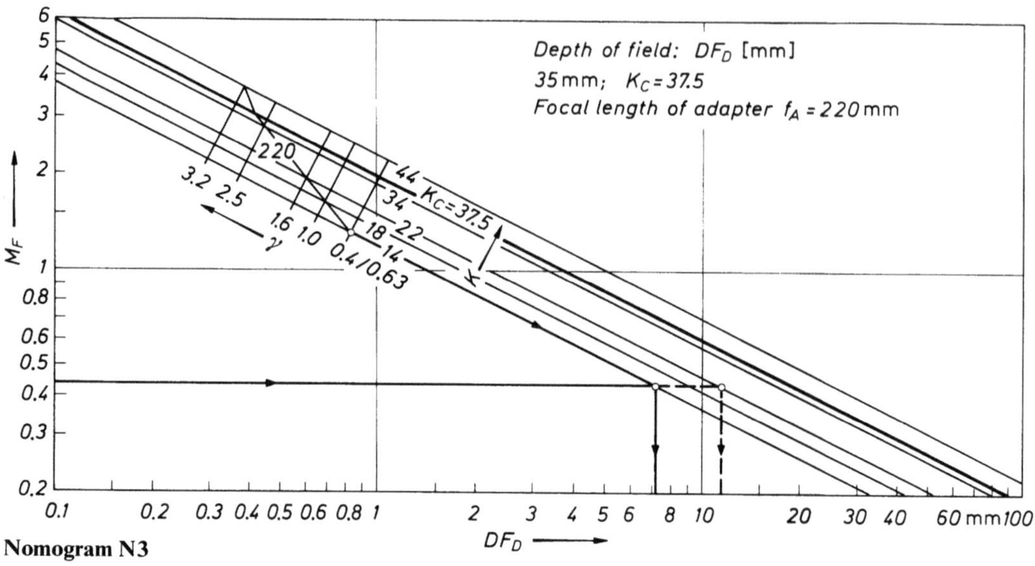

Nomogram N3

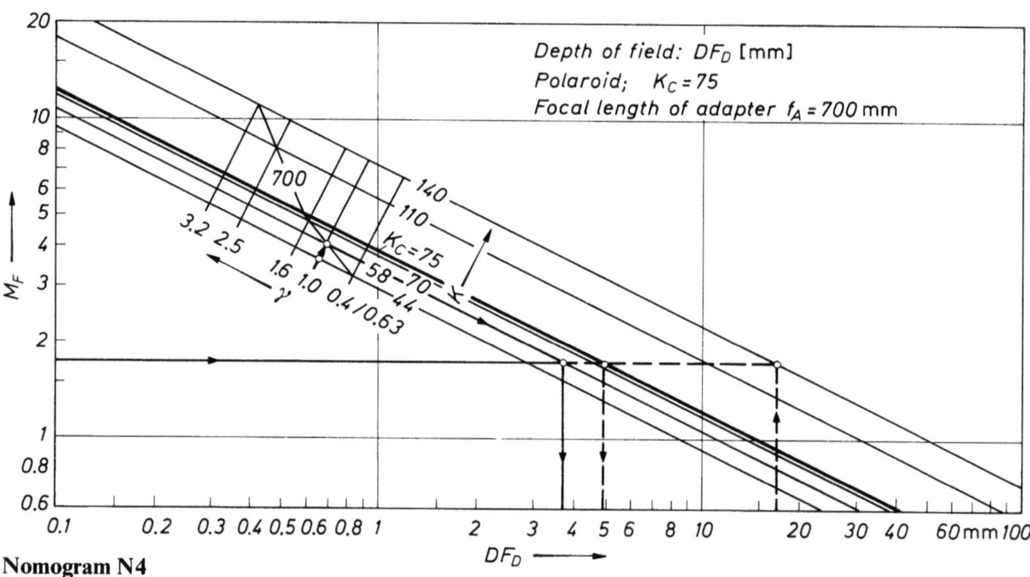

Nomogram N4

Documentation is carried out with the photo adapter $f_A = 220$ mm on 35 mm format ($U = 0.05$).

According to nomogram N3 the point of intersection of magnification changer curve 0.4 and adapter curve 220 yields $K_{min} = 14$.

The value of $M_F = 0.44$ is taken from nomogram 1. The depth of focus $DF_D = 7.2$ mm is taken from the intersection of $M_F = 0.44$ and $K = 14$. As said before, this also guarantees optimum resolution. The useful f/number being $K_C = 37.5$, there is no unsharpness due

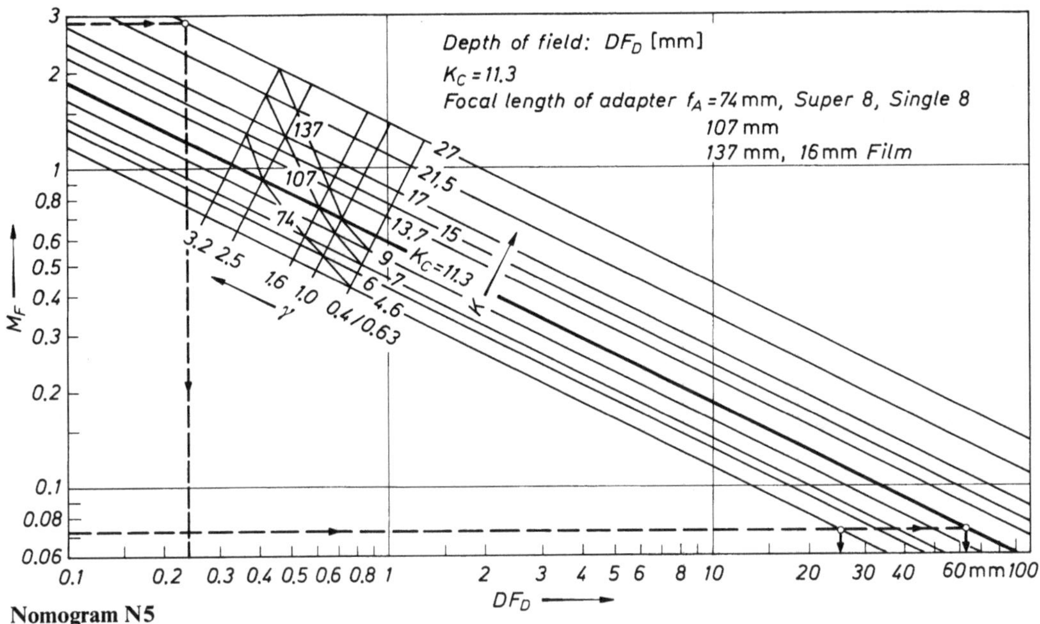

Nomogram N5

to diffraction. For a greater depth of focus under otherwise equal conditions, e.g. DF_D = 11.5, $K = 22$ must be set on the f/number dial. There will be no unsharpness due to diffraction, but the object-side instrument aperture will be smaller, and the resolving power not fully utilized.

Second example: an operation microscope with $f_O = 400$, $\gamma = 1$ and Polaroid adapter yields according to nomogram N4 in the point of intersection of adapter and magnification changer curves $K_{min} = 58$. With the value $M_F = 1.75$ taken from nomogram N1, $DF_D = 3.8$ mm. The useful f/number $K_C = 75$. This guarantees full resolution. With $K_C = 75$ (dotted horizontal line) full resolution is maintained, but the depth of focus can be increased to $DF_D = 4.9$ mm (dotted vertical line). $K = 140$ would have to be set for $DF_D = 17$ mm, but on account of a loss in resolution. Nomogram N5 is used similar to the other two nomograms.

10.7 Illumination intensity in the film plane

10.7.1 Coaxial illumination

The following equation applies to the illumination intensity E_F in the film plane:

$$E_F = B_C \cdot \frac{1}{f_O^2 \cdot K^2}$$

where B_C is a constant, f_O the focal length of the primary objective and K the f/number.

For a certain adapter type the illumination intensity in the film plane is only dependent upon the primary objective and the magnification of the Galilean changer or zoom system. As said before, the latter determines the f/number K.

The following recommendation results from this relationship: documentation should be carried out with the shortest possible focal length of the primary objective. Low magnification of the changer or zoom system should be used because then the f/number is the smallest. It also minimizes irradiation of the operating field.

10.7.2 Oblique illumination

In the case of oblique illumination the following equation applies to the illumination intensity in the film plane:

$$E_F = B_O \cdot \frac{1}{K^2}$$

where B_O is a constant.

There is no dependency on the objective focal length. With given K only the specific properties of the oblique illumination enter the equation.

10.8 Stereopsis

Stereopsis is the capability to recognize depth differences in binocular vision. Schober, for instance, discusses the theoretical principles in detail.

The depth perception (not to be confused with the depth of focus) is dependent upon the stereo angular resolving power α which is connected with the vernier visual acuity. It depends on the brightness in the object space and amounts to about 10 angular seconds for daylight vision.

For an operation microscope the depth perception is determined by the following equation:

$$\vartheta = \frac{\alpha \cdot f_O^2}{a \cdot \gamma \cdot \Gamma_T \pm \alpha \cdot f_O}$$

where a is the distance between the two changer or zoom axes, Γ_T the magnification of the tube lens/eyepiece combination (Fig. 143). Because the product $\alpha \cdot f_O$ is negligible with respect to $a \cdot \gamma \cdot \Gamma_T$, it follows that

$$\vartheta = \frac{\alpha \cdot f_O^2}{a \cdot \gamma \cdot \Gamma_T} \, .$$

It is interesting to compare the depth perception of an unaided eye with that of an operation microscope. In the first case the distance eye/object is assumed to be 250 mm ($\hat{=} f_O$), the pupil distance $a = 65$ mm, and $\gamma \cdot \Gamma_T = 1$.

It then follows that $\vartheta = 0.045$ mm.

An operation microscope consisting of a primary objective $f_O = 250$ mm, a paired Galilean magnification changer $\gamma = 0.63$ at a distance $a = 22$ mm, a tube $f_T = 125$ mm, and a 10× eyepiece has a depth perception of $\vartheta = 0.042$ mm, which is comparable with the one above.

The depth perception can be considerably improved if the magnification changer is set to position $\gamma = 2.5$. It then follows that $\vartheta = 0.011$ mm, which gives a much better three-dimensional impression of the object. As a matter of fact, the depth perception is the better the smaller ϑ.

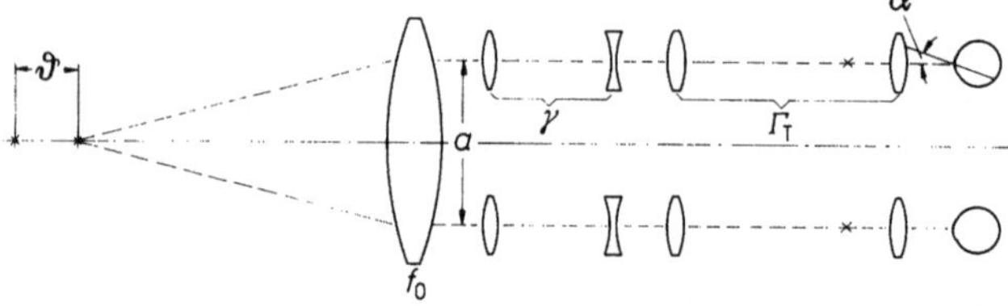

Fig. 143. Stereopsis.

Literature

1. Barraquer, J.; Littmann, H: El microscopio para filmar Modelo Barraquer – Zeiss. An. Inst. Barraquer *8*, 227–236 (1968)

2. Barraquer, J. I.; Barraquer, J.; Littmann, H.: A new Operating Microscope for Ocular Surgery. Am. J. Ophthalmol. *63*, 90–97 (1967)

3a. Berek, M.: Grundlagen der Tiefenwahrnehmung im Mikroskop. Sitzungsberichte der Gesellschaft zur Förderung der gesamten Naturwissenschaften zu Marburg *62*, 189–223 (1927)

3b. Berek, M.: Zur Theorie der Abbildung im Mikroskop. Optik 5, 1–30 (1949)

4. Flügge, J.: Leitfaden der geometrischen Optik und des Optikrechnens. Göttingen: Vandenhoeck u. Ruprecht 1956

5. Françon, M.: Einführung in die neueren Methoden der Lichtmikroskopie. Karlsruhe: Braun 1967

6. Harms, H.; Mackensen, G.: Augenoperationen unter dem Mikroskop. Stuttgart: Thieme 1966

7a. Jakubowski, H. G.; Riedel, H.: Der Motorkopf zur elektrischen Vertikalbewegung des Operationsmikroskops. Zeiss-Inf. *63*, 34 (1967)

7b. Jakubowski, H. G.; Riedel, H.: Zusatzeinrichtungen für das Operationsmikroskop nach Barraquer: Das Mitarbeitermikroskop und der Adapter zur Querverstellung des Spaltbildes. Zeiss-Inf. *74*, 132–133 (1969)

8a. Littmann, G.; Wittekind, R.: Operationsmikroskop mit neuer Photoeinrichtung und neuem Mitbeobachtertubus, Zeiss-Inf. *58*, 149–153 (1965)

8b. Littmann, G.; Riedel, H.; Jakubowski, H. G.: Mitarbeitertubus und Film-(Fernseh-)Adapter für Zeiss Operationsmikroskope. Zeiss-Inf. *75*, 5–12 (1970)

9a. Littmann, H.: Ein neues Operationsmikroskop. Klin. Monatsbl. Augenheilkd. *124*, 473–476 (1954)

9b. Littmann, H.: Ein neues Operationsmikroskop mit Photoeinrichtung. Naturwiss. Rundsch. *9*, 391–393 (1954)

9c. Littmann, H.; Ein neues motorisiertes Operationsmikroskop für die Mikrochirurgie des Auges. Klin. Monatsbl. Augenheilkd. *153*, 99–106 (1968)

9d. Littmann, H.: Operating microscopes for ocular microsurgery. An. Inst. Barraquer *9*, 299–325 (1969)

9e. Littmann, H.: Zwei neue motorisierte Operationsmikroskope mit physiologisch angepaßter Vergrößerungssteuerung. Klin. Monatsbl. Augenheilkd. *157*, 61–65 (1970)

9f. Littmann, H.; Riedel, H.: Zwei neue Operationsmikroskope. Klin. Monatsbl. Augenheilkd. *160*, 221–223 (1972)

10. Riedel, H.; Jakubowski, H. G.; Sümmerer, G.: Das Mitarbeitermikroskop und die Operationslupe. Zeiss-Inf. *79*, 63–64 (1972)

11. Schober, H.: Das Sehen, Bd. I, 4. Aufl. 1964; Bd. II, 3. Aufl. 1970; Leipzig: VEB Fachbuchverlag

Subject index